BEHAVIORAL ASPECTS IN DENTISTRY

BEHAVIORAL ASPECTS IN DENTISTRY

Barbara D. Ingersoll, Ph.D.
Associate Professor
Department of Behavioral Medicine
Department of Community Dentistry
West Virginia University
Morgantown, West Virginia

Appleton-Century-Crofts / **New York**

82 83 84 85 86 / 10 9 8 7 6 5 4 3 2 1

Prentice-Hall International, Inc., London
Prentice-Hall of Australia, Pty. Ltd., Sydney
Prentice-Hall of India Private Limited, New Delhi
Prentice-Hall of Japan, Inc., Tokyo
Prentice-Hall of Southeast Asia (Pte.) Ltd., Singapore
Whitehall Books Ltd., Wellington, New Zealand

Library of Congress Cataloging in Publication Data

Ingersoll, Barbara D., 1945–
    Behavioral aspects in dentistry.

    Includes index.
    Contents: An overview of behavior dentistry—
Communication skills and relationship enhancement—
Special problems in communication—[etc.]
    1. Dentistry—Psychological aspects. I. Title.
[DNLM: 1. Dentistry—Psychology. 2. Dentist-
Patient relations WU 61 I47b]
RK53.I53   617.6'001'6   81-12676
ISBN 0-8385-0631-3   AACR2

Text design: Piedad Palencia
Cover design: Piedad Palencia

PRINTED IN THE UNITED STATES OF AMERICA

To my parents, Frederick and Jean Sahl

CONTRIBUTORS

JAMES BENNETT, D.M.D.
Hospital Dental Service
University of Oregon Health Sciences Center
Portland, Oregon

ASUMAN KIYAK, Ph.D.
Department of Community Dentistry
University of Washington
School of Dentistry
Seattle, Washington

J. WILLIAM ROBBINS, D.D.S.
San Antonio Veterans Administration Hospital
  and Department of Restorative Dentistry
University of Texas Dental School
San Antonio, Texas

JOHN D. RUGH, Ph.D.
Departments of Restorative Dentistry and Psychiatry
University of Texas Dental School
San Antonio, Texas

DORIS J. STIEFEL, D.D.S., M.S.
Department of Oral Medicine
Dental Education for Care of the Disabled
School of Dentistry
University of Washington
Seattle, Washington

D. ELOISE STULL, M. Ed.
Department of Rehabilitation Medicine
University Hospital
University of Washington
Seattle, Washington

CONTENTS

CHAPTER 10

APPENDIX

PREFACE

Among health care professionals, the dental profession has long been in the vanguard in seeking ways to reduce anxiety, minimize pain, and motivate patients to comply with health care recommendations. Such problems, our colleagues in dental practice assure us, are far more numerous and troublesome than the dental student or young dentist might suspect.

Issues of dentist-patient interaction and patient management have received considerable attention in the dental curriculum in recent years and, at the same time, an increasing number of behavioral scientists have directed their efforts toward research programs designed to shed new light on these old problems.

This book draws upon the results of research in behavioral dentistry for assistance with patient management problems frequently encountered by the practicing dentist. Of course, many questions remain to be answered, but we believe that the groundwork has been laid for a scientific approach to the study of patient management problems in dentistry.

Many colleagues have provided invaluable assistance in the preparation of this book. I am particularly grateful to Drs. Rick Seime and Bill McCutcheon, and to Dean Robert Biddington for their enthusiastic support. I am also indebted to Drs. Eric Jackson and Don Kruper for their painstaking reviews and many useful suggestions. Loreen Hurley was, as usual, calm through many a minor crisis and capably organized a million scribbled slips of paper into a coherent manuscript. Special thanks are owed to Marcia Kipnees, who recognized the need for this text; to Liz Stueck, who encouraged me to persevere; and to my husband, Tom, my *primum mobile* in all respects.

BEHAVIORAL ASPECTS IN DENTISTRY

An Overview of Behavioral Dentistry

For many years, dental educators emphasized the development of technical expertise and stressed the study of basic sciences and mastery of manual skills. Although the dental profession as a whole has long been characterized by a concern for "the person behind the teeth," few dental schools provided programs of instruction in the sociocultural and interpersonal aspects of dentistry.

Recently, however, an increased focus on these important factors has led to changes in dental education. The scope of the behavioral sciences within dentistry has expanded, interest has been sparked in such areas as disease prevention and community health, and new content areas have emerged.

One such new area concerns the behavioral aspects of dental practice. We refer to this field as "behavioral dentistry," a term which emphasizes the importance of understanding human behavior for the practice of dentistry. Patricia Bryant, of the National Institute for Dental Research, has proposed the following definition of behavioral dentistry.[1]

> Behavioral dentistry is the interdisciplinary field concerned with the development and integration of behavioral and biodental science knowledge and techniques relevant to oral health and disease, and the application of this knowledge and these techniques to prevention, diagnosis, treatment, and rehabilitation.

Topics of particular concern in this field include:

- the dentist–patient relationship and communication styles and patterns which enhance this relationship

- the reduction of fear, pain, and stress
- promoting patient compliance with treatment instructions and oral hygiene and dietary recommendations
- management of the fearful or uncooperative child patient
- correction of maladaptive oral habits, such as bruxism and the exaggerated gag reflex

Dental students—especially those in the first or second year of dental school—sometimes ask, "Why a course in behavioral dentistry? We need to learn technical skills—besides, teeth do not 'behave.'"

In reply, we point out that, when asked to describe problems with which they are confronted as practitioners, few dentists mention deficiencies in technical skills—their own or those of other dentists.[2] It would seem that dental schools do a commendable job of providing students with technical expertise.

The practicing dentist, however, must be more than a technician of the oral cavity; for, while teeth do not "behave," they are attached (more or less firmly) to people and, in his dealings with the people who are his patients, the dentist must assume a number of diverse roles. He must, for example, function as a businessman and manager if he is to earn his livelihood in his profession. The dentist is also an educator who provides his patients with information concerning preventive activities and persuades them to carry out these activities. In this role, the need for good communication skills is obvious. The ability to communicate effectively is essential, too, in explaining treatment plans and giving posttreatment instructions. Finally, the dentist must have special skills to deal with special patients—fearful patients, patients in pain, the handicapped, the elderly, fearful or uncooperative children and their anxious parents.

The skills demanded of the dentist are many and varied in these multiple roles. It is in conjunction with these roles, rather than in the role of oral technician, that the dentist most frequently reports encountering problems.

PROBLEMS: THE DENTIST'S PERSPECTIVE

Problems encountered by the practicing dentist were investigated in a recent national survey.[3] A sample of over 500 practicing dentists responded to a list of problems by checking those encountered in their practices. The results of this survey are presented in Table 1-1.

Although some of the problems listed in Table 1-1 are clear-cut business management problems (insurance paperwork, scheduling patients) and are therefore outside the scope of behavioral dentistry, most of the problems cited are clearly behavioral in nature. The frequency with which these prob-

TABLE 1-1. BUSINESS AND PATIENT MANAGEMENT PROBLEMS REPORTED BY A NATIONAL SAMPLE OF PRACTICING DENTISTS*

Problem	% Reporting Problem (N = 589)	% Ranking Problem Among Most Important
Fear	87.4	26.5
Broken, cancelled, late appointments	76.0	30.9
Not motivated for oral hygiene	76.0	36.2
Do not follow treatment instructions	74.7	17.7
Fee collection	72.3	31.9
Insurance paperwork	69.6	28.7
Ignorant of benefits of preventive care	69.2	28.7
Disruptive or uncooperative children	59.4	4.6
Dentist's lack of business knowledge	55.0	30.4
Explaining treatment	45.6	11.5
Parents	39.0	2.5

* From Ingersoll, Ingersoll, McCutcheon, and Seime, 1979.

lems were reported is consistent with previous research showing that, although dentists consider most of their patients to be pleasant, considerate people who pay their bills, they report encountering problems with about 20 percent of them.[4]

As Table 1-1 indicates, fear is the most commonly encountered patient management problem. Fear is a principal reason for dental avoidance, which is estimated to affect about five to six percent of the adult population, or approximately 11 to 13 million people.[5] In Chapter 4 we will describe the origins of dental fear and discuss methods for reducing such fear. Pain, an important source of dental fear, is discussed in Chapter 5.

Fear is also an important factor in broken or cancelled appointments, a problem reported by over three-quarters of the dentists surveyed. Patients who arrive late for appointments, cancel with little notice, or simply fail to appear for an appointment play havoc with the dentist's schedule—and managing a dental schedule is, at best, much like performing a juggling act. The schedule must have a minimum of costly "down time," yet it must be flexible enough to accommodate patients who require emergency treatment. Patients, of course, want appointments suited to their schedules, which further complicates the process. It is not surprising that over half of the dentists surveyed reported problems with scheduling.

Patients who seem poorly motivated to follow oral hygiene recommendations were cited as a problem by over three-quarters of the dentists surveyed. A comparable number cited patients who do not follow treatment instructions, and over two-thirds reported problems with patients who, seemingly ignorant of the benefits of preventive care, seek help only on an emergency basis or demand extractions when restorative procedures could be performed. Such patients are a source of considerable frustration to the practitioner, who knows that the incidence of dental caries and periodontal disease could be drastically reduced through preventive activities. However, despite large-scale educational programs and the often heroic efforts of individual practitioners, the public has shown little interest in prevention, and it is small wonder that dentists view the public as lax, unmotivated, and emergency oriented.[6]

Patients who do not pay their bills are, understandably, a source of considerable concern to the dentist. This problem is not limited to low-income areas, nor is it restricted to those in a particular dental specialty: As Table 1-1 indicates, almost three-quarters of the dentists surveyed reported this problem. On the surface, this might appear to be a straightforward business problem. However, research suggests that when such a situation arises, it is often the dentist–patient relationship which is at fault. When the relationship between patient and caregiver is characterized by mutual trust and respect, the patient is more likely to pay his bills and to do so promptly. Additional benefits of a good dentist–patient relationship are described in Chapter 2, as are communication skills, an essential component of a good relationship.

Over half of the dentists surveyed reported problems with child patients. In fact, it has been estimated that the average dentist in general practice sees one to two children each week who present behavior problems in the operatory.[7] The uncooperative or fearful child presents special problems in the dental context. Not only does disruptive behavior interfere with the dentist's attempts to provide care in an efficient manner; it also increases the likelihood that the child will experience pain. Further, memories of early difficulties and unpleasant experiences can sow the seeds of later fear of dentistry.[8]

Not infrequently, the dentist encounters problems with the parent as well as with the child. Parental anxiety, overprotectiveness, or harsh disciplinary measures undertaken in the reception area or operatory can have adverse effects on child behavior during the dental visit. Problems of pediatric management have been the focus of a good deal of research, from which many helpful suggestions and strategies have emerged. These issues are considered in Chapter 7.

PROBLEMS: THE PATIENT'S PERSPECTIVE

Just as dentists report encountering problems with their patients, so do patients register complaints about dentists and dental treatment. Although not all of the problems about which patients complain are readily amenable to change, many arise as a result of misunderstandings and a lack of awareness on the part of the dentist and his staff. Attempts to minimize or avoid such problems are in the dentist's own best interest, as satisfaction in his professional role is closely related to the satisfaction of his patients with the service they receive.

The attitude of the public toward dentists and dentistry can be assessed through a number of channels. Interestingly, attitudes expressed through one channel are not always consistent with those expressed through other channels. For example, one measure of the public's perception of dentistry is the stream of jokes, cartoons, television programs, and even movies in which dentists are portrayed as merciless sadists and dental treatment depicted as a unique form of torture. Paradoxically, however, when asked to rank various professions according to prestige, the public rates the prestige of the dentist high, placing him above the pharmacist, lawyer, hospital nurse, and school teacher.[5]

When attitudes based on personal experience with dentists are assessed, people tend to be more consistent. It is heartening to note that most people report reasonable satisfaction with the dental care they have received. One large-scale study reported that the public evaluates the dentist on the basis of quality of dental work, the dentist's personality and way of relating to people, his concern about causing pain, and his fees.[9] The authors concluded that, "On the whole . . . most persons seem satisfied with the degree to which (these) criteria are met." In fact, in a recent survey conducted for the American Dental Association, 63 percent of the respondents who had visited a dentist in the last year said that they had never been dissatisfied with the care they received.[10] Further, 81 percent said they would strongly recommend their dentist to friends.

However, these surveys also show that approximately one-third to one-quarter of the respondents reported an unsatisfactory experience or an experience which gave them less confidence in dentists. Specific complaints included poorly executed, ineffective, or unnecessary treatment; painful treatment; inconsiderate, rough, or unfriendly manner; and high fees. Unexplained high fees were also cited in another survey of patient complaints.[11] Other problems included officious, overbearing office assistants; assembly-line practices; and lengthy waits in the waiting room. Additional evidence of patient dissatisfaction with dental care is the high rate of patient turnover within the individual practice. It is estimated that dentists have a 50 percent turnover of patients within a five-year period and that over half of this attrition can be attributed to patient dissatisfaction.[12]

Finally, malpractice claims have become a problem of some significance. Dental malpractice suits are increasing rapidly—perhaps even more than in the case of medicine—and the cost of dental malpractice insurance is rising accordingly.

Experts agree that, as in medicine, most malpractice suits stem from problems in the patient–professional relationship, rather than from technical error. One states:

> Since 90 percent of doctors who are sued are not guilty of technical error, and since many doctors who are guilty of known error are not sued by their patients, we must look at the doctor–patient relationship for the major causes of claims and suits.[13]

Some patients sue to avoid paying fees which they consider unjustified. Others bring suit to obtain revenge for what they perceive as unfair or impersonal treatment. Suits also arise when the patient holds unrealistic expectations concerning treatment outcome—expectations which can sometimes be encouraged inadvertently by the overly enthusiastic or optimistic professional.

A psychological profile has been developed of the patient most likely to sue. Such a patient is described as "dependent, emotionally immature, extreme, rigid and authoritarian, incapable of accepting adult responsibility, and quick to suspect and to blame others for his frequent troubles."[14]

Characteristics of the professional most likely to be sued have also been identified. The suit-prone professional cannot admit, to his patients or to himself, his own limitations and inabilities. As a consequence, he fails to warn patients of potential problems and finds it difficult to seek assistance from colleagues when it might be necessary and appropriate to do so. Faced with a dissatisfied patient, the suit-prone professional refuses to discuss the problem. Instead, he tries to avoid the situation by avoiding the patient until, finally, he is forced to deal with both in a court of law.

DENTISTRY'S INHERENT HANDICAPS: PAIN, COST, AND INVASION OF SPACE

In addition to the specific areas of difficulty described in the preceding sections, still others exist which, at this time, are intrinsic to the practice of dentistry. These factors—pain, cost, and invasion of the patient's personal space—are a source of strain in the dentist–patient relationship and constitute handicaps under which virtually every dentist must work.

Pain

Dentists have been in the vanguard in their constant search for more effective ways to reduce pain and promote patient comfort. Yet, despite dramatic technological and pharmaceutical advances which have greatly reduced the amount of pain associated with dental treatment, some degree of pain or discomfort still accompanies most dental procedures.

Pain is very closely related to dental fear and avoidance. In one large group of patients who described themselves as fearful, almost half cited pain as the reason[15]; among patients who had not visited a dentist for a year or more, ten percent said they feared the pain involved in dental work.[10]

How painful is dental treatment? In general, pain associated with dental treatment is rated as milder than other types of clinical or laboratory-induced pain, including cancer and back pain. Most patients rate pain associated with dental treatment as greater than "no pain," with average ratings falling somewhere between "no pain" and "somewhat painful."[16]

As one authority notes, these findings do not suggest that dental treatment is painless.[16] But he adds, it is not surprising that many dentists may view their work as painless, since fearful patients (who are less apt to tolerate pain well) are not likely to seek care regularly. Thus, the dentist's "typical" patient is likely to be a "good responder"—that is, one who considers dental pain only mildly annoying.

The dentist must remember, however, that even among these patients, pain is experienced, although what pain is felt is not likely to be reflected in body movements, facial expression, complaints, or other easily detected behavior. It is also important to remember that the discomfort may not end when the patient leaves the operatory but may persist for hours or even days after certain procedures.

Cost

In the recent ADA survey cited in a previous section, 23 percent of those who had not visited a dentist for a year or more gave high cost as the major reason. As in all areas of health care, the cost of service delivery in dentistry is high. Many patients simply cannot afford good oral health care. As it seems unlikely that dental care will be included in a national health care program, the cost of care will remain an insurmountable obstacle for many people.

Even among affluent individuals, the cost factor cannot be dismissed. The decision to undergo expensive treatment may mean postponing other, more immediately enjoyable purchases, such as a new car or a vacation. For many, this is a difficult choice, especially if they are not experiencing pain or discomfort at the time.

Invasion of Personal Space

Territoriality, the tendency to lay claim to and defend a territory, has been extensively studied in animals. It is not uncommon for animals to risk injury or even death defending their territory against invasion. Well known, too, are the deleterious effects of overcrowding on animal health and behavior.

Man, too, engages in territorial behavior. "Territory" usually refers to a specific geographic area or piece of land, but there is also a kind of "portable" territory we carry around like invisible bubbles. This zone of distance between the self and others, called "personal space," is an important but often overlooked variable in interpersonal relations.

Social norms govern the use of personal space. These norms vary with different cultures and, within a culture, with age, sex, and status. Women, for example, stand closer together than do men, children closer than adults, and friends closer than strangers. Distinct zones in which different kinds of social interactions occur have been identified within our culture.[17] These range in distance from the public zone (approximately 12 to 25 feet), the distance used for public lectures, to the intimate zone (touch to one and a half feet), the distance reserved for interaction between lovers and between parents and children.

It is within this latter area, the intimate zone, that dental treatment takes place. Thus, dental treatment, by its nature, involves violation of the patient's personal space.

Although we absorb and observe the norms of our culture concerning personal space without conscious awareness, when these norms are violated people react with discomfort and sometimes even with violence. When their space is invaded, people communicate discomfort by body language. These communications range from subtle movements to attempts to leave the area. If escape is prevented and the invasion continues, the person may become hostile and may even aggress against the intruder.

Fortunately, although many patients fidget in the dental chair, few actually flee and even fewer assault the dentist. However, it is important for the dentist to remember that his work involves a violation of the patient's personal space and to bear in mind the degree of discomfort this can produce.

TOWARD A BRIGHTER FUTURE

The problems described in the preceding sections highlight the conflict that can occur between dentist and patient and suggest the need for change. Change is needed in the form of new strategies to reduce fear and to manage chronic and acute pain; better methods of persuading patients to comply with oral hygiene recommendations; improved methods of communicating with patients—in short, devising new ways of managing the patient problems described in the preceding sections.

A firm foundation for such change can only be provided by careful scientific investigation. It is puzzling that in a field such as dentistry, in which new methods and materials are subjected to rigorous tests before they are adopted for clinical use, the same standards have seldom been applied to methods and techniques which relate to human behavior.

To date, however, little of what has passed for behavioral science in dentistry has, in fact, been very scientific in nature. Unsupported speculations have been advanced as established facts; anecdotes and accounts of personal experience have been far more common in the dental literature than reports of controlled experiments.

Much of the material which has appeared in the dental literature concerning human behavior reflects the popularity of psychodynamic, or Freudian, thought. Psychodynamic theory emphasizes the importance of difficult or traumatic early experiences, repressed impulses, and unconscious processes in human behavior.

Thus, dentists have been told that negative attitudes toward dentistry often result from unconscious conflict within the patient's personality. This conflict is thought to stem from problems encountered by the patient during the "oral stage," which occurs during the first 18 months of life. Psychodynamic theory holds that difficulties during this early period can result in a patient who, as an adult, views dental treatment as an attack. For such a patient, invasion of the oral cavity represents a frightening threat to psychological well-being. Fear of dentistry has been variously described by psychodynamic theorists as fear of mutilative retaliation for unacceptable impulses, fear of loss of control over one's own impulses, and projection of the patient's aggressive impulses onto the dentist, who the patient then fears as a dangerous aggressor. It has also been speculated that the noncompliant patient has trouble in his relationships with authority figures and that the bruxer is attempting to repress hostile impulses.

These speculations are certainly fascinating but, since we have stressed the importance of scientific evidence, it is reasonable to ask: Do research findings support these theories? Does the evidence support the notion of a relationship between personality variables, such as hostility, and observable dental behavior? In fact, very little research has actually been undertaken on this topic. Of the few studies that have appeared, none has supported a clear-cut relationship between personality variables or repressed impulses and dental behavior.

More importantly, however, psychodynamic theory does not lend itself readily to practical application in the dental office. Although the dentist may find psychodynamic theory interesting and provocative, he cannot turn to this literature for direct assistance with practical, everyday problems of patient management.

A model, or theory, of human behavior which appears to have more immediate practical implications for dental practice is the behavioral approach. Behavioral psychology offers an alternative explanation for the origins of attitudes and behavior—dental as well as nondental. According to behavioral theory, the origins of a person's attitudes, beliefs, and behavior do not lie in repressed impulses or in unconscious fears or desires. Instead, we should look to the person's life experiences and learning history for the sources of his current attitudes and behavior. In short, behaviors and beliefs are learned and people behave as they do because they have learned to do so.

This view leads us to expect that early unpleasant dental experiences might lie at the root of fear of and avoidance of dentistry in adult life. Further, as people learn by observing the behavior of others, we might predict that patients whose friends and family are fearful of dental treatment will, themselves, be fearful patients. As we shall see, results of recent research support these hypotheses. An additional advantage of the behavioral model is that it stresses overt behavior rather than unconscious impulses or personality variables. Repressed impulses and personality traits are difficult to define and impossible to observe directly. For this reason, it is difficult to examine them scientifically and to pose questions which can be investigated through research. Overt behavior, however, can be defined and observed with greater ease. Thus, researchers can more readily test hypotheses and questions derived from the behavioral model and find answers backed by experimental evidence.

Within psychiatry and psychology, the behavioral approach has produced excellent results. New treatment methods have been developed for a broad range of human problems. These methods have been carefully researched and many have been shown to be far more effective than other treatment methods previously employed.

Recently, researchers have begun to apply this approach to patient management problems in dentistry. Systematic, well designed programs of research, many of them funded by the National Institute for Dental Research, have shed new light on old problems.

These studies, which represent the initial steps toward a science of behavioral dentistry, form the basis of this book. In the following chapters, this research is presented and implications for the dental practitioner are discussed. New methods are described in detail to help you, the practitioner, employ them correctly and successfully. The merits and drawbacks of each are examined so that you can make informed decisions about the suitability of a particular method for your own use.

Each of the techniques to be described has been shown to be effective. We believe that these methods, if appropriately used, can aid in patient management and significantly reduce problems and conflict between the dentist and the people who are his patients.

REFERENCES

1. Bryant, P. S. "Behavioral dentistry: Concept and challenge." In *Clinical Research in Behavioral Dentistry: Proceedings of the Second National Conference on Behavioral Dentistry,* edited by B. D. Ingersoll and W. R. McCutcheon, pp. 1–8. Morgantown, W. Va.: West Virginia University Press, 1979.

2. Ingersoll, T. G.; Ingersoll, B. D.; Seime, R. J.; McCutcheon, W. R. "A survey of patient and auxiliary problems as they relate to behavioral dentistry curricula." *J Dent Educ* 42:260, 1978.
3. Ingersoll, B. D.; Ingersoll, T. G.; McCutcheon, W. R.; Seime, R. J. "Behavioral dimensions of dental practice: A national survey." Unpublished manuscript, West Virginia University School of Dentistry, 1979.
4. Weinstein, P.; Milgrom, P.; Ratener, P.; Read, W.; Morrison, K. "Dentists' perceptions of their patients: Relation to quality of care." *J Pub Health Dent* 38:10, 1978.
5. Friedson, E. and Feldman, J. "The public looks at dental care." *Am Dent A J* 57:325, 1958.
6. Rayner, J. F. "Communication between the public and the dental profession." *Am J Pub Health* 63:21, 1973.
7. Weinstein, P. "Identifying patterns of behavior during treatment of children." In *Clinical Research in Behavioral Dentistry: Proceedings of the Second National Conference on Behavioral Dentistry,* edited by B. D. Ingersoll and W. R. McCutcheon, Morgantown, W. Va.: West Virginia University, 1979, p. 115.
8. Kleinknecht, R. A.; Klepac, R. K.; Alexander, D. K. "Origins and characteristics of fear of dentistry." *Am Dent A J* 86:842, 1973.
9. Kreisberg, L. and Treiman, B. R. "Dentists and the practice of dentistry as viewed by the public." *Am Dent A J* 64:806, 1962.
10. American Dental Association Bureau of Economic and Behavioral Research. *Dental Habits and Opinions of the Public: Results of a 1978 Survey.* Chicago, Ill., 1979.
11. Hellman, V. "Eight reasons why your patients won't be back." *Dent Econ* 62:22, 1972.
12. Collett, H. A. "Dental malpractice: An enormous and growing problem." *J Prosth Dent* 39:217, 1978.
13. Editorial: "Breakdown in doctor–patient relationship is shown by malpractice suits, say psychologists in C.M.A. study." *Am Col Sur Bul* 44:137, 1959.
14. Blum, R. H. *The Management of the Doctor–Patient Relationship.* New York: McGraw-Hill, 1960.
15. Kleinknecht, R. "Fear of dentistry: Its development, measurement and implications." In *Advances in Behavioral Research in Dentistry,* edited by P. Weinstein, Seattle, Wash.: University of Washington, 1978.
16. Klepac, R. K. "The role of pain in dental apprehension." In *Clinical Research in Behavioral Dentistry: Proceedings of the Second National Conference on Behavioral Dentistry,* edited by B. D. Ingersoll and W. R. McCutcheon. Morgantown, W. Va.: West Virginia University, 1979, p. 52.
17. Hall, E. J. *The Silent Language.* New York: Doubleday, 1959.

2

Communication Skills and Relationship Enhancement

There is considerable evidence suggesting that a good relationship between dentist and patient is a necessity rather than an option or an "extra." Because the average patient is not able to assess accurately the technical competence of his dentist, he must judge him by other standards. In most cases, he bases his judgment on the dentist's interpersonal skills—the extent to which the dentist shows understanding, respect and concern for the patient.

In the previous chapter, we noted some of the problems which can arise when the caregiver–patient relationship is poor. We now turn to the benefits which accrue to both you and your patients when this relationship is characterized by mutual trust and respect. Many authorities for example, have directly linked the placebo effect to the quality of the caregiver–patient relationship. There is general agreement that the placebo effect is an important component of all medical and dental treatment and of all medications— even a drug as potent and pharmacologically active as morphine. Thus, the quality of the dentist–patient relationship can actually have significant effects on treatment outcome.

Other benefits, too, have been identified.[1] When the relationship between caregiver and patient is good, we find that:

- the patient is more likely to remember and follow instructions
- the patient is more likely to pay his bills on time
- the patient speaks highly of the professional and recommends him to others
- the patient shows significant anxiety reduction
- the patient is less likely to sue

We think that when these points are considered, the value of a good dentist–patient relationship is quite clear. The obvious question now becomes, "How can I develop such a relationship with my patients?"

We are sometimes asked about the feasibility of teaching relationship skills. Many believe that the development of a good chairside manner comes only with years of experience. Others confuse good relationship skills with that elusive quality, "charm," and maintain that it cannot be taught: one is either mysteriously blessed with charm or must muddle through without it. Still others maintain that good patient management requires only common sense.

Certainly, experience is important. As a young dentist gains experience, he becomes more assured in the professional role. As he gains confidence, he can focus less on his own anxiety and more on the needs of his patients. In this respect, there is no substitute for experience.

Experience also provides the opportunity for a dentist to learn through trial and error. However, trial and error is not a particularly efficient approach to learning, as each new learner must, in effect, reinvent the wheel. Further, experience alone does not ensure that one will eventually acquire the most effective skills. Consider the golfer who slices the ball: unless he corrects his swing, years of golfing will result only in a very well-rehearsed slice.

Thus, we do not argue with the need for experience. We do, however, believe that students can learn basic skills which, with practice, will greatly enhance their ability to interact with patients and to develop mutually satisfying dentist–patient relationships.

As concerns so-called "common sense," we believe that it is often not sufficient to deal effectively with the problems health care professionals encounter. What, for example, is the "common sense" way to tell a patient that he has a terminal illness? In such a situation, it is sensitivity rather than common sense that is needed. Can sensitivity be taught? The term "sensitivity," like "charm," really refers to a particular group of verbal and nonverbal behaviors that most people interpret as evidence of interest, concern, and caring. It is possible to identify many of these behaviors and to specify their components with some precision. With practice, the average student is capable of mastering these skills and using them successfully, as considerable research has shown.[2] The essentials of communication skills are discussed in detail in the following sections.

CHARACTERISTICS OF FACILITATIVE COMMUNICATION: WARMTH, EMPATHY, AND RESPECT

The basis of a successful dentist–patient relationship lies in the dentist's ability to communicate effectively with his patients. Communication occurs at an emotional level as well as at a cognitive or intellectual level. In the dental setting, it is often the emotional or feeling level which is more important. As a dentist, you must communicate to your patients that you are concerned; that you consider them and their problems important; and that you will listen and will make a genuine effort to understand their feelings and points of view.

Note that we do not say that you will be able to solve all of the patient's problems; this, of course, is not possible. Health professionals are often confronted with problems for which there are no solutions—problems such as chronic illness and death. Because we can, by virtue of our training and expertise, provide solutions to some problems, we can easily fall into the trap of believing that we should have the power to solve all problems. When we are faced with problems for which there is no solution, we often become uncomfortable and, in our discomfort, seek to avoid interacting with the person. This is especially unfortunate, because it is the person with an unsolvable problem who most needs to know that others will at least listen and care.

Successful and effective communication is characterized by three core qualities: *warmth, empathy,* and *respect.* Considerable research has shown that professionals who communicate with high levels of warmth, respect, and empathy are rated as more effective on measures of social, personal, and vocational functioning.[3] Communication which embodies all of these characteristics is called *facilitative communication,* because it facilitates interpersonal interaction. It makes it easier for people to discuss problems, understand the important feelings involved, and arrive at satisfactory solutions.

Warmth

When we communicate warmth, we communicate an interest in and a concern for the other person. Warmth is communicated primarily through nonverbal behaviors, such as head nodding, eye contact, appropriate facial expression, and other nonverbal signs of interest and attention.

Eye contact is an especially important component of warmth. Lack of eye contact is most often interpreted as lack of interest. Thus, the dentist who asks a patient, "How are you today?" while standing with his back to the patient, washing his hands, or checking his instrument tray, conveys that he really doesn't care about the answer to this question. To avoid conveying this unfortunate impression, it is best to attend to such tasks before the patient enters the operatory. If this is not possible, greet the patient, then excuse yourself to engage in the necessary activity. A good rule of thumb is: address the patient only when you are prepared to devote your full attention to his reply. Otherwise, you might miss subtle but important signals and cues to his emotional state.

The thoughtful dentist will also remember to introduce his assistant to the new patient. Although this involves verbal rather than nonverbal behavior, we mention it in this section because this behavior demonstrates a concern for the patient's overall comfort. It is awkward and embarrassing for the patient to have to address the assistant as "Uh."

Some practitioners attempt to build rapport and put the patient at ease by engaging in chit-chat about the weather, sports, and the like. While this is appropriate in an ordinary social situation, it is important to remember that the dentist–patient relationship is not a social relationship but a professional one. We believe that rapport is best established by showing a real interest in the patient and the problems that bring him to your office.

Communicating warmth does not mean behaving in a gushy fashion. Effusive, "buddy-buddy" behavior typical of the used-car salesman is not necessary or desirable. If you have a real commitment to understanding your patients and a genuine concern for their well-being, warmth will usually be conveyed in a natural fashion.

Empathy

Empathy—the attempt to perceive and understand a situation from the point of view of another person—is usually considered the most important characteristic of facilitative communication. To empathize with another person means to try to stand in his shoes and to look at the world through his eyes.

Note that empathy differs from sympathy, which means pity or compassion. Sympathy can also mean "sameness of feeling," as "I am in complete sympathy (agreement) with you on that point." Empathy, on the other hand, denotes an attempt to understand the other's feelings, even when they are very different from your own.

Empathic communication builds up the other person. It conveys the message, "I care enough about you to try to understand your feelings and your point of view."

Respect

We use the word "respect" to mean an awareness that others are entitled to have feelings and perceptions which are different from our own. Respect implies the realization that no one holds a monopoly on absolute truth; that others have a right to view things differently from the way in which we do.

Note that respect does not necessarily imply agreement. To respect the right of another person to view the world differently is merely to acknowledge that he does have that right. Indeed, it is inevitable that each individual have his own perception of a situation: each, after all, has a unique genetic background, learning history, and assortment of abilities and disabilities. All of these factors interact in a complex fashion to determine how an individual views and responds to a situation. To insist that others see the world exactly as we see it is, at best, naive and, at worst, arrogant.

One of the most common ways in which lack of respect is communicated is by giving advice. As one authority points out:

> Think for a moment about the last time someone gave you advice. . . . Was the advice something you hadn't already thought of? Did you use that advice? Would you have been just as well off if you hadn't been given that advice? We suspect that many times you have felt insulted by inappropriate, worthless advice that has been given to you, even when it was given with good intentions. Most of us have given thoughtless advice, without realizing that when we do this, we are saying, "Any simple thing that I think of off the top of my head is better than what you have thought of, even though you have been thinking about this matter for a long time."[4]

"But," you are probably wondering, "what about dental advice? What about advice concerning oral hygiene and preventive care? What about recommendations for treatment? What about all the oral health care problems on which patients seek our advice?"

It is very important to distinguish between giving advice and giving information. The statement, "If you do not have this restorative procedure done, you will probably lose that tooth," is information. The dentist draws on his special knowledge and provides the patient with facts to which he, the dentist, has access but the patient does not.

On the other hand, consider the following: "If I were you, I would certainly have the work done now. Surely you can't think that buying a new car is more important than taking care of your teeth!" This statement constitutes advice. It is an attempt to make a decision for the patient that only he can make. You may consider teeth more important than cars, but the patient's decision must be based on his value system not yours—they are, after all, his teeth.

It is, of course, perfectly appropriate and quite important to educate your patients, to make them aware of the facts concerning oral health, and to teach them the skills to maintain good oral health. However, it is not appropriate to become angry or upset if the patient does not act as you think he should: to do so will alter little except your own blood pressure.

In the following examples, compare advice with information.

EXAMPLE A

Patient: My wife complains that I'm spending too much money on this treatment.

Dentist: Tell her that you'll quit spending so much money on your teeth if she quits spending so much at the beauty parlor.

Comment: This statement constitutes advice. Unless the dentist has been trained as a marriage counselor, he would do well to avoid telling patients how to manage their spouses.

EXAMPLE B

Patient: Do I have to have all of the work done right away? This is a busy time of year at the plant and it's hard to get away.

Dentist: Those front teeth need immediate attention to stop the decay. The other work can be done over the course of the year.

Comment: The dentist has provided the patient with enough facts about his oral condition to enable the patient to make an intelligent, informed decision about treatment.

Giving advice is only one way in which lack of respect is communicated. You also communicate lack of respect for the other person when you:

1. Argue with the other person about the facts of the matter.

Patient: Your receptionist was really rude to me on the telephone.

Dentist: Oh, I'm sure she didn't mean to be rude. You must have misinterpreted.

Comment: Even if you believe that the other person is misinformed or mistaken, it is unwise to begin by arguing with him. First, listen to the other person. Then, when he is sure you have understood his point of view, you can present the situation from your point of view.

2. Pass judgment on the feelings or perceptions of the other person.

Patient: I'm so depressed about wearing dentures. I feel like an old hag.

Dentist: Now, that's silly. You know you'll look better—and you'll be able to chew your food better, too.

Comment: When you tell the other person that his feelings are foolish or bad, you imply that the person himself is foolish or bad for feeling as he does.

3. Minimize or dismiss the other person's feelings in an attempt to make him feel better or reassure him.

Mother of young patient: No, I don't want to wait in the reception room. I can't just leave my baby in here all alone!

Dentist: Now, don't worry about a thing. We'll get along just fine.

Comment: Telling another person, "It's not that bad," or "Don't worry" is seldom helpful. You are not a magician. You cannot make the other person feel better simply by telling him to feel better. That doesn't make the feelings disappear—it just makes the other person stop talking to you about them. That may make you feel better, but it does little or nothing to help the other person.

EMPLOYING FACILITATIVE COMMUNICATION

Communications that are empathic and respectful convey to the patient that you consider him important enough to try to understand how he feels. Of course, before you can convey understanding of how another person feels, you must be able to identify the feelings, whether they are explicit and overtly stated ("I'm just furious about this bill"), or only implied by such cues as tone, inflection, and facial expression. To do this, you must listen very intently not only to what is said but also to how it is said.

Impediments to Careful Listening

To put aside your own feelings and to listen to what the other person is really saying is a difficult task which demands your full attention. It is a particularly difficult task because it is so different from the way in which we usually interact with others. In social situations, we have learned to listen with only a portion of our attention. While another is speaking, we are usually thinking about what we will say when it is our turn to speak.

Attending only to what the other person is saying is an especially difficult task for health care professionals. Dentists and doctors tend to listen only to that which might be helpful in formulating a diagnosis and treatment plan because we equate helping with doing something, saying something, taking some action. Often, especially when there is no action that will be helpful, simply listening to the patient is the most helpful thing a health professional can do.

External events are one source of distraction which can interfere with careful listening. This is especially true in a busy dental office where there are many demands on the dentist's attention.

The greatest impediment to careful listening, however, is usually the listener's own feelings. The listener may feel helpless and uncomfortable when the patient expresses sadness or grief, embarrassed when he discusses personal matters, and defensive toward the angry or critical patient. Because these emotions interfere with the ability to listen attentively and perceive accurately, they are impediments to clear communication. We discuss some of the ways in which the dentist can deal with his own emotional responses in later sections.

Reflective Responding: Getting the Message Across

It is not sufficient simply to be aware of the patient's feelings and to understand his point of view; this awareness and understanding must be directly and clearly communicated to the patient. At the simplest level, understanding is expressed by nonverbals such as nodding the head and by phrases such as "Um hm," and "Yes, I see."

The most powerful and direct means of communicating understanding is a method known as *reflective responding*. The term "reflective," as it is used here, means "mirrorlike"; the listener serves as a mirror, reflecting back to the patient the attitudes and feelings he has expressed.

The Purpose   This method was originally developed for use in psychotherapy to communicate the therapist's understanding and acceptance of the patient's feelings, emotions, and attitudes. However, you do not have to be a psychologist or a psychiatrist to use this method successfully. Nor, in fact, should you restrict your use of reflective responding to communicating with your patients. All people — your staff, your colleagues, even your family and friends — feel good when someone shows enough concern to listen and to understand.

This, then, is the primary purpose of reflective responding: to communicate the message, "I am listening; I understand." This message is perhaps the single most important ingredient in a sound relationship between patient and professional.

Reflective responding serves another important function in the dental context. This method of communicating focuses the attention of both dentist and patient on the patient and his problems and thereby prevents the dentist from slipping into the role of the patient's adversary. In an earlier section we cautioned against arguing with the patient about the facts of the matter, passing judgment on his feelings, and minimizing or dismissing his feelings. Each time you do — indeed, any time you contradict, disagree, or voice an opinion which differs from that held by the other person, even if you do so with tact and courtesy — you assume an adversarial position relative to that person.

Of course it would be a dull world if no one ever disagreed with anyone else, and we do not suggest that this is an appropriate goal. However, disagreement presents special problems in the dentist–patient relationship, because feelings of antagonism can develop to the great detriment of the relationship. The step from adversary to antagonist is not a large one, but once taken, it is very difficult to reverse.

When antagonism develops between dentist and patient, the dentist may find himself defending his authority and expertise. The wise dentist will never permit this to occur. He knows that, by virtue of his training and knowledge, he is the expert. To defend his position is not only unnecessary, it is also the surest way to undermine it.

Reflective responding offers an effective way to avoid these potential problems. By focusing on the patient's feelings and demonstrating a desire to understand, the dentist can prevent unnecessary disagreements which profit neither dentist nor patient.

The Process The process of reflective responding can be described very simply. To use reflective responding: 1) Listen and observe to identify the attitudes and feelings expressed by the other person; 2) Restate, in your own words, these feelings and attitudes.

If, for example, the speaker's tone of voice and facial expression indicate that he is angry, the listener reflects this feeling by saying, "That situation really made you mad," or "You're pretty angry about that." Similarly, if the speaker indicates that he feels sad or sorrowful, the listener reflects these feelings.

A complete reflective response includes reference to the feelings the speaker expresses and to the situation causing these feelings. The formula, "You feel A (*describe emotion*) because B (*describe situation*)" may be useful to help you remember the components of a reflective response. Study the examples of reflective responding below.

EXAMPLE A

Patient: I try my best to take care of my teeth like you showed me, but all you ever do is criticize me.

Dentist: It makes you angry that you try so hard and I don't show any recognition of your efforts.

EXAMPLE B

(*Pedodontist has just explained nursing bottle caries to the mother of a young patient*)

Mother: But, Dr. Hendricks, what can I do? I can't just let him cry. I'd feel awful!

Dentist: You feel bad when he cries—you worry that you're not a good mother.

EXAMPLE C

> Patient: I'm not going through with any more treatments. I've spent too much time and money already.

> Dentist: Progress has been slow and you're feeling fed up with the whole thing.

The process of reflective responding may seem insultingly simple. However, students are often surprised to find that when they attempt to practice reflective responding, it is actually rather difficult at first because it runs counter to long-standing habits of responding to content, not feelings. Frequently, problems arise as a result of incorrect use of the word "feel" in the formula, "You feel A because B." If "feel" is used to mean "think" or "believe," the resulting response will relate only to content, not feelings. Compare the following examples.

EXAMPLE A

> Dentist: Mr. Fredericks, I'm a little puzzled. I know that my assistant taught you the proper way to brush and floss, but I'm afraid I don't see any improvement yet. Is there some problem?

> Patient: I know I should do those things but, you know, I've been so busy lately that I just haven't been able to find the time.

> Dentist A: You feel that you have been too busy to brush and floss regularly.

> Dentist B: Maybe you feel a little bit resentful—like I don't understand your busy schedule and I'm making unreasonable demands.

> *Comment:* Dentist A makes no reference to the patient's feelings. In this case, the patient probably feels trapped and under some pressure to come up with an excuse. Dentist B's response is a reflective response.

EXAMPLE B (*Dentist has just explained treatment plan and fees.*)

> Patient: Your fees are outrageous! How do you expect me to pay for this treatment?

> Dentist A: You feel my fees are too high.

> Dentist B: It's distressing that the treatment is so expensive. Perhaps you wonder, too, whether it's really going to be worth it.

> *Comment:* The patient doesn't "feel" the fees are too high, he *thinks* the fees are high. He *feels* distressed and upset because a deci-

sion to go ahead with the treatment will involve some sacrifice and he is not sure it will be worth such sacrifice. (Note: This example also illustrates the patient who, when worried, frustrated, or otherwise upset, behaves in an angry fashion toward the dentist—see section on "The Angry Patient." Reflective responding can be especially helpful in "de-fusing" such situations, whereas defensive responding from the dentist can lead to escalation and conflict.)

The beginner may find, too, that it is initially somewhat difficult to respond reflectively without sounding like a parrot or a broken record. To avoid this hazard, paraphrase, using your own words.

Patient: (*Describing pain of recent onset*) I'm worried sick about it. I hope I'm not going to lose any teeth.

Dentist A: You're worried about the pain. You hope you're not going to lose any teeth.

Dentist B: It's frightening when you don't know what's causing the pain. You tend to suspect the worst.

Comment: Dentist A just repeats what the patient has said. Dentist B paraphrases, with better results.

Common Questions   Students often comment that reflective responding, as described in the brief examples above, doesn't "go anywhere"; it doesn't solve the problem. Of course, the flavor of reflective responding cannot be adequately conveyed in such brief examples. Extended examples in the next section will help you understand how reflective responding often helps the patient find his own solution to a problem. However, in this context, it is important to repeat a point made earlier: patients will often present you with problems you do not have the power to solve. In such situations, you can be of greatest help by listening and conveying your understanding and concern.

Below are some other questions students commonly ask about reflective responding.

Q: With a busy practice, how can I find time to listen to all of my patients?

A: Reflective responding can actually save time because clear communication leads to fewer misunderstandings and fewer problems with dissatisfied patients. Actually, reflective responding requires more effort than time, but in those cases in which it is necessary to spend additional time with a patient, it is perfectly legitimate to charge for your time, just as you must charge higher fees for other time-consuming procedures.

Q: How can I distinguish between a situation in which I should respond reflectively and one in which I should simply provide information?

A: In general, reflective responding is helpful in any situation in which the patient expresses emotions, feelings, or attitudes. Certainly, there are times when it is not appropriate to use reflective responding. If, for example, someone asks, "Is it cold out?" you would not say, "You are curious about the weather." But be careful: questions are not always simple requests for information. They can also be used to express a variety of feelings. The patient who asks, "Do you think my mouth will ever be in good shape?" may be expressing frustration; the patient who asks, "Have you done this procedure often?" may be asking, "Can I trust you to do the job well?" For this reason, questions can be traps. Compare the following and note the difference between the two situations.

EXAMPLE A

Patient: My husband is picking me up after my appointment. What time will we be finished?

Comment: Simple request for information.

EXAMPLE B

Patient: (*Tensely*) What are you going to have to do today? Will it take very long? When will we be finished?

Comment: This patient is anxious. Reflection of feelings would be appropriate.

Q: What should I do if I am not sure how the speaker feels?

A: This situation can be handled by being tentative in your reflective response. You might ask, "Are you saying . . . ?" or "You mean . . . ?" to indicate your uncertainty. If you are wrong, the patient will correct you and is likely to appreciate your efforts to understand, even when they are not completely successful.

Q: Suppose the speaker expresses conflicting feelings?

A: Because people are so complex, a person may express two very different emotions or attitudes at the same time. When this is the case, the listener should reflect all the feelings expressed. A patient may say, for example, "I get so tired of these treatments—although I guess they really are helping me." In such a case, reflect both feelings—frustration and feeling better—without praising the positive feelings or criticizing the negative ones. Patients are especially likely to have mixed feelings when anger is one of their emotions. If they are allowed to express their angry, negative feelings openly, positive feelings often follow.

EXTENDED INTERACTIONS

This section might be appropriately subtitled, "What Do You Say After You've Said 'You feel Anxious'?" After an initial introduction to reflective responding and some brief examples, students are often confused. "Where does it lead?" they ask. "Do I just keep reflecting everything the patient says? I can just see it: at five o'clock, I'll still be there with my one o'clock patient, reflecting his feelings!"

Reflective responding is used to establish a relationship and to identify problems and areas of difficulty. After a few cycles in which the patient speaks and the dentist responds reflectively, the typical dentist–patient interaction reaches one of several outcomes. These outcomes are shown in Figure 2-1.

Frequently, the outcome falls clearly into Categories A, B, or C as shown in Figure 2-1. Category A refers to situations in which the problem has been clearly identified, but the problem is one for which there is no readily available solution. This category includes a very broad range of real-life events, ranging from rain on a picnic to loss of a spouse. Again, we stress the importance of listening. Avoid the temptation to offer platitudes or glib reassurance. Instead, listen and, through listening, provide emotional support.

In Category B are those situations in which the problem has been identified as the patient's need for information or instruction. You may have just discovered that your patient uses a side-to-side movement when brushing his teeth and requires instruction in the proper technique. Or your patient

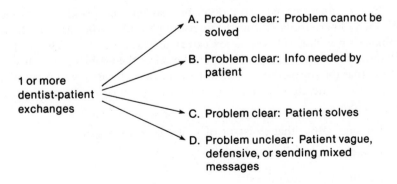

FIG. 2-1. Possible outcomes resulting from initial dentist–patient exchange.

may ask, "When can I chew on that side?" or "Is there a particular brand of toothpaste that's better than the others?". In such situations, your task is clear: provide the necessary information and/or instructions and check to be sure the patient has understood.

Many times, the outcome falls into Category C: the problem has been clearly identified and the speaker has either provided his own solution or has otherwise indicated that he can deal with the situation. The following is an example.

Receptionist: (*Obviously annoyed*) Dr. Jensen, I've really had it with the way Mrs. Conners lets her kids run all over the waiting room. They're so noisy—and what a mess they make!

Dentist: It's pretty upsetting to you when they run around like that. You're worried, too, about how much they might annoy the other patients.

Receptionist: Yes, they're like wild Indians. I wouldn't mind the noise so much if they would just stay in the play area.

Dentist: It's the running around that really bothers you. If you could figure out a way to keep them in the play area, you'd feel more comfortable, even if they were a little noisy.

Receptionist: Yes. We couldn't tie them up, could we? (*Laughs*) Well, you know, my sister is a teacher and she was telling me about a gold-star system she uses to reward good behavior in her class-room. I wonder if something like that would work for us.

Dentist: Great idea. We could even use "prizes" if they earn so many stars.

Receptionist: OK, I'll talk to my sister. She can help me figure out the details.

In the situations we have described so far, the problem was clearly identified. There is also a fourth outcome possible—the case in which the problem is not clear. This situation can arise in several ways. Often a patient will indicate that he has a problem, but he states the problem in such a vague fashion that the problem is not clear to you. In such cases, you must be very specific and concrete if you are to elicit enough information to understand the problem.

Patient: Boy, that assistant of yours is really a pain.

Dentist: Miss Henderson annoys you?

Patient: She sure does!

Dentist: I'd like to hear more about that. Does she do anything in particular that annoys you?

Patient: She's just stuck-up.

Dentist: Stuck-up? You think she's been rude or unfriendly toward you?

Patient: Yeah, she acts funny.

Dentist: Funny?

Patient: She just acts like she doesn't like me.

Dentist: That must be upsetting to you. Can you tell me what she does that seems unfriendly?

Patient: Well, she doesn't talk to me. She just ignores me, like I'm not even here.

Further questioning reveals that the assistant, busy with preparations, did not hear the patient speak to her and so did not respond. When this is explained to the patient, he accepts the explanation and seems content. The dentist privately reminds the assistant to excuse herself when she leaves the patient's side to attend to other tasks.

Sometimes difficulty in identifying a problem arises because the patient is defensive and shows reluctance to discuss a particular topic, such as his oral hygiene practices, the medication he is taking, or feelings of anxiety which the dentist has detected. The defensive patient often behaves in a fashion which others interpret as hostile. Such patients are usually not angry; rather, they are anxious. This is understandable: Patients take a risk when they disclose private material—the risk that they will be rejected, scorned, belittled, or ridiculed. They are worried, uncomfortable, and uncertain as to how you will respond. These feelings, then, are the ones you reflect to the patient.

- It's hard for you to talk about this.
- Perhaps you are concerned about what I might think of you.
- You wonder if I really need this information.
- You feel like I am intruding on your privacy by asking all these questions.

Research has shown that an effective way to help a person provide information about a topic he considers potentially embarrassing is to model, or demonstrate, such self-disclosing behavior for the patient. If, for example, you have been in a similar situation in which you found it difficult to talk or provide needed information, you might share this with the patient.

- I'm sort of a private person and I feel reluctant to give information when I'm not sure why the other person needs to know. Perhaps if I explained why I need this information, you might feel more comfortable.
- I had to wear braces when I was in high school and I remember feeling pretty upset about it at times. Sometimes I used to get angry with my dentist because he didn't seem to understand how I felt.
- I found flossing my teeth an awful nuisance at first, too. I had trouble remembering to do it regularly, and then I would worry that my dentist would yell at me or criticize me for forgetting.

On occasion, difficulty in identifying a problem arises when the patient or speaker sends conflicting messages. There may, for example, be a discrepancy between the patient's verbal behavior and his nonverbal behavior, as in the case of the patient who says, "I'm perfectly relaxed," while clenching his hands into fists. Or there might be a discrepancy between what the patient says and what he does, as in the case of the patient who says, "I'll do anything to get better," yet fails to comply with treatment and medication recommendations.

Pointing out such discrepancies to the patient carries an element of risk. Unless the relationship is firmly established, the health care professional takes a chance that the patient will perceive him as harsh and judgmental. If you decide to take such a risk in the interest of providing good care, inform the patient of the perceived discrepancy in a straightforward, nonjudgmental fashion. The purpose of confrontation is simply to provide the patient with another view of the situation, it is not an opportunity to play "Gotcha!"

EXAMPLE A

Results of an exam indicate that the patient has new areas of decay; the dentist has explained this to the patient.

Patient: More work! I'm really sick of getting bad news every time I come in for a checkup.

Dentist: You couldn't be that sick of it or you'd start to take better care of your mouth.

Comment: This response is judgmental and likely to make the patient feel defensive.

EXAMPLE B (*same situation*)

Dentist: It upsets you that on each visit we find more decay.

Patient: It sure does. Just once, I'd like to come in for a checkup and hear, "No problems. Everything's fine."

Dentist: That puzzles me. When I examine your mouth, I see that you're not very regular in your home care. Yet you say you really want good checkups.

Comment: The dentist points out a discrepancy between what the patient says and what he does without conveying blame or criticism.

By calling the patient's attention to specific discontinuities in his behavior, you can help him deal with areas of conflict to which he has not previously attended. If this is done tactfully, it can be a helpful means of resolving a problem.

REFERENCES

1. Bates, R. C. *The Fine Art of Understanding Patients.* Oradell, NJ: Medical Economics Book Division, 1968.
2. Runyon, H. L. and Cohen L. A. "The effects of systematic human relations training on freshman dental students." *Am Dent A J* 8:196, 1979.
3. Carkuff, R. R. *Helping and Human Relations: A Primer for Lay and Professional Helpers.* Vol. 1. New York: Holt, Rinehart and Winston, 1969.
4. Gazda, G; Walters R; Childers, W. *Human Relations Development: A Manual for Health Sciences.* Boston: Allyn and Bacon, 1975.

3

Special Problems
in Communication

The principles of good communication discussed in Chapter 2 can help you build sound relationships with most of your patients. Some patients, however, pose a special challenge and to manage these patients competently, special skills are required. This "handle-with-care" group includes patients who are angry and hostile, those who are depressed, and a sizable number who are fearful of dental treatment.

THE ANGRY PATIENT

Most of us would probably admit to some difficulty in dealing with the patient who is angry, hostile, or critical. In fact, even professional counselors who have been especially trained to deal with "difficult" patients often react negatively to the hostile patient.[1]

How do dentists typically react to the hostile or critical patient? In a recent study, dentists were asked for their responses to a patient who was highly critical of her previous dentist and to a patient who complained about the cost of treatment.[2] In dealing with such patients, respondents tended to reply in a defensive fashion. ("I'm sure your last dentist knew what he was doing.") Others tried to reason with the patient, offering logical arguments to show that the fee was reasonable or the previous dentist was competent; that it was the patient who was incorrect or at fault. Unfortunately, such tactics—which amount to little more than arguing with the patient—are seldom helpful in disarming a hostile patient.

Among health professionals, other common responses include responding with placating and conciliatory behavior in an attempt to smooth over the situation as quickly and quietly as possible and—worse—respond-ing with counter hostility. The former response—attempting to placate the patient—is unsatisfactory because it sweeps the problem under the rug. Unfortunately, problems treated in this fashion seldom remain buried but usually emerge again at a later date or in a different guise. Unless problems are openly discussed, they will remain unresolved and a threat to the profes-sional–patient relationship.

Responding with hostility is obviously even less satisfactory. It sets in motion a cycle of hostility–counterhostility which can be destructive to the patient and which leaves the professional feeling ashamed and guilty.

You cannot deal effectively with the emotionally upset, angry patient if you become upset, defensive, or angry yourself. Before we discuss methods for responding helpfully to the angry patient, we will first suggest an ap-proach to keeping your own emotions under control.

Dealing with Your Own Emotions

Think back to the last time you were harshly criticized or verbally attacked by an angry person. How did you feel? Perhaps you felt a little shaken and experienced unpleasant symptoms of physiological arousal. Maybe you be-came upset and defensive and tried to argue with the angry person. Or per-haps you found yourself becoming angry and shouting back.

We realize that it can be very difficult to remain calm and accepting when you are confronted with anger and hostility. Strong emotions are contagious and spread quickly from one person to another.

Of course strong emotions do have survival value in the face of real danger. The physiological arousal that accompanies strong emotion pre-pares the individual to flee the attacker or fight to defend himself. Seldom, however, do we face the danger of a real physical attack. As we noted ear-lier, few patients, no matter how angry, actually hit their dentist. Yet even when there is no real likelihood of bodily harm, we respond as if there were. We perceive criticism and anger as an attack and respond with arousal and defensiveness.

This response pattern probably originates in childhood, when a par-ent's anger can signal a spanking and the hostility of peers and siblings is often accompanied by overt physical aggression. Through the repeated pairing of anger with pain, we associate the anger of others with harm to ourselves. We learn to respond to all indications of anger as if they were actual physical attacks.

This response pattern, including physiological arousal, occurs so quickly that it seems almost automatic. An event takes place and, like the knee jerk reflex when the knee is tapped, a corresponding emotion occurs in response. Most people consider their own role as rather passive and view themselves as simply experiencing the emotions that some person or event has caused to occur. Our language reflects this common view. We say, for example, "That made me mad," or "He hurt my feelings," as if we were merely passive victims of external manipulation.

However, although emotions develop quickly, they do not occur instantaneously, nor are they automatic. Human beings do not possess built-in switches which can be directly triggered by external events to produce emotional responses. The development of an emotional response is not a simple two-stage process in which an event leads to an emotion. An emotional response is more appropriately viewed as the result of a three-stage process: (1) an *event* occurs; (2) the individual *perceives* and *thinks about* the event; and (3) the individual *experiences* the physiological and subjective components of an emotion.

As an example of this process, consider the following:

Event: Patient says, "This treatment hasn't helped me a bit. Are you sure you know what you're doing?"

Thoughts: Dentist thinks, "He's implying that I'm incompetent. How awful of him to say that. I won't stand for it!"

Emotional Response: Dentist feels upset, aroused, angry.

As you can see, what a person thinks or tells himself about an event determines how he will respond emotionally to the event itself. If he tells himself, "This is awful, terrible, outrageous," the result will be a strong negative emotion. If, however, he merely tells himself, "This is inconvenient," or "This is an unfortunate nuisance," he avoids strong negative emotions at Point 3.

Unfortunately, most of us are in the habit of telling ourselves some rather silly things about events that happen to us. As a consequence, we often experience unpleasant emotional upset.

Can we do anything to correct this habit? Albert Ellis, founder of the Institute for Rational Living and author of many books for professional and lay readers, argues that, indeed, we can correct the things we say to ourselves and can, thereby, spare ourselves needless unpleasant emotional upheavals. Ellis states that our emotion-producing "self-talk" can be corrected by examining and actively challenging the irrational assumptions and beliefs on which it is based. These irrational beliefs, which we probably acquire during childhood, include such notions as: "It is a dire necessity for me to be liked by everyone with whom I come in contact; it is horrible if someone doesn't like me or think well of me," and, "I should be absolutely competent in everything I undertake, especially if the task is important to me. It is a catastrophe if I make a mistake."

We don't argue that it is preferable to be liked and respected by others.

When people are generally well-disposed toward us, it makes life easier and more pleasant. But is it a dire necessity that we be liked and respected by everyone? Is it really awful, horrible, unthinkable if someone is angry or critical?

Similarly, it isn't enjoyable to make mistakes, especially if the consequences are fairly serious. But we are, after all, only human and human beings are inevitably fallible—it's part of being human.

Unless the other person is actually threatening physical assault, it is simply not logical or rational to become upset and angry at his words. We smile condescendingly at the belief of some primitive tribes in the magical power of words, calling their incantations "mumbo-jumbo." But is our behavior any more rational when we respond with anger and perhaps even violence to being called an unpleasant name? The old jingle, "Sticks and stones can break my bones, but names can never hurt me" makes very good sense. Words cannot hurt us—unless, of course, we tell ourselves that they can.

When you are attacked by an angry or critical person, the first step is to examine your own "gut" response. If you find yourself becoming anxious or angry, ask yourself, "Why do I think it's so terrible that this person is angry or that he thinks I am less than perfect? Am I really so fragile that an angry or critical word can destroy me?"

Remember, if you feel angry with your unreasonable, hostile, or difficult patients, it is because you are telling yourself, "How dare this person behave like this! This is atrocious! It's an outrage and I won't stand for it!" If, on the other hand, you tell yourself firmly (and you will have to be firm with yourself, because anger is a habit that is difficult to break), "This is simply an unfortunate nuisance," you can avoid making an unpleasant situation even worse for all concerned.

Identifying the Source of the Anger
When confronted with an angry or critical patient, you cannot respond effectively until you have answered this question: Why is this person angry? This question is often overlooked, but it is crucial to an understanding of the patient and his problem.

It is important to remember that the other person's anger might have little to do with anything you have said or done. You might be simply a handy target for anger that is really directed toward someone or something else or even toward the angry person himself. We have all been guilty of misdirecting angry and hostile feelings. Spouses, children, the family dog are all perceived as "safe" outlets for our pent-up emotions and are often the targets of misplaced anger.

Because patients view the dental assistant and the receptionist as lower in status than the dentist and, therefore, "safer" to attack, displaced anger is likely to be directed toward them rather than toward the dentist. The anger that the patient feels toward the dentist who has kept him waiting or who has sent a bill that seems too high is often expressed in the patient's interactions with the dentist's employees. Of course, it is important for the dentist to help his assistants learn to respond to such attacks in a calm, nonhostile fashion. Otherwise, the situation quickly becomes a major problem for the dentist.

Another underlying cause of angry, hostile behavior is fear. Many people cannot admit to themselves or to others that they are fearful. They deal with feelings of anxiety and helplessness by expressing their fear as anger, lashing out at others to mask their true feelings. This is especially likely to happen when a person is ill or in pain. Even the most placid, good-natured person can become irritable and edgy when illness occurs.

Anger and irritability are sometimes symptoms of depression. Suggestions for recognizing and helping the depressed patient are presented in the next section.

Unrealistic expectations are often a source of unwarranted anger directed at health care professionals. Many patients endow the dentist and the physician with magic powers because, as one authority[3] has noted:

> . . . they do not know the nature and limitations of medical knowledge. When the magic is ineffective or takes longer than anticipated, the patient may react with disproportionate or inappropriate anger and recrimination.

As we noted in an earlier section, malpractice suits can arise when the patient holds unrealistic expectations concerning treatment outcome or when he is not aware of problems which might accompany or follow the treatment. To protect himself and the patient, the dentist must be very sure that he and the patient agree on expectations concerning treatment outcome, time course, and potential risks involved.

This is particularly important in specialty areas such as orthodontics and prosthodontics, where unrealistic expectations may be more frequently encountered than in other specialties or in general practice dentistry. In fact, at least one orthodontist, Doctor Julian Singer,[4] recommends using an informed consent form with all patients. After diagnosis, treatment plan, and possible complications and sequelae are explained to him, the patient signs a consent form outlining his responsibilities in the treatment process and risks involved in treatment. Doctor Singer adds that, far from frightening patients out of the decision to proceed with treatment, his explanations and consent forms have "generated positive interest and have not deterred acceptance of treatment."

There is one final factor to consider in assessing the source of a patient's anger. It is entirely possible that the patient's criticism is grounded in fact; perhaps the dentist really has made an error or has kept him waiting for quite a while. Dentists are not, as we have noted, above human failings and fallibility.

Whatever the reason for the patient's anger, there is only a single method for identifying that reason and that is to listen to the patient. Let the angry person talk. Encourage him to talk. An angry person expects you to put up a fight, to defend yourself, or to become angry in return. The quickest way to disarm him is to show a real interest in his problem and his feelings. Such an interest indicates to the patient that you are on his side, and it is difficult to remain very angry with someone who responds with interest and understanding. Phrases which communicate this interest include:

- You sound very angry. Would you like to tell me about it?
- I can see you're really very annoyed. Is there anything I can do to help?
- You seem pretty upset with me. I'd like to hear more about it.

Remember that anger interferes with the ability to think clearly and to perceive accurately. The angry person is likely to be illogical. Do not try to argue with him or reason with him while he is upset. When angry feelings are consistently recognized and reflected, they tend to be followed by more positive feelings. Only then is the person able to analyze the problem rationally.

The following examples illustrate interactions between a dentist and an angry, upset patient. In comparing these examples, notice that the first dentist falls into the trap of defensiveness. The second dentist avoids this trap, with much better results.

EXAMPLE A

Dentist: I'm afraid there's no doubt about it, Mr. Anderson. There is recurrent decay under that crown. We'll have to remove it.

Patient: Remove it? When you put this crown on, you told me it would last for years and years.

Dentist: And it would have—if you had cared for your teeth properly.

Comment: The dentist responds defensively, blaming the patient for the problem. While the problem might, indeed, be the patient's fault, blaming an angry patient for his problem will probably be perceived by the patient as a counterattack.

Patient: Cared for my teeth! That's what I pay you for!

Comment: The patient becomes even less rational as he grows angrier. It is obvious that he feels that his dentist has let him down. The dentist would do better to address these feelings directly.

Dentist: Mr. Anderson, I can't go home with you to make sure you take care of your mouth. There's just so much I can do.

Comment: The dentist continues to avoid the patient's feelings. Instead, he tries to reason with the patient. Reasoning, however, is seldom effective with an angry person. In addition, it usually sounds defensive and argumentative.

Patient: Well, "just so much" turns out to be not enough. You told me this crown would take care of this tooth. It didn't—and now I expect you to make good on it.

Comment: This conversation could easily turn into a shouting match, with the patient storming out of the office to seek the services of another dentist—or even an attorney.

EXAMPLE B

Dentist: I'm afraid there's no doubt about it, Mr. Anderson. There is recurrent decay under that crown. We'll have to remove it.

Patient: Remove it? When you put this crown on, you told me it would last for years and years.

Dentist: You're really shocked. You thought that you were pretty well set. Now you find out that we're back to the beginning again and you're pretty angry.

Comment: The dentist does not become defensive. He acknowledges and accepts the patient's feelings.

Patient: I certainly am! Wouldn't you be?

Comment: When patients ask, "Wouldn't you feel the same way?" or "How would you feel?" they are really asking, "Try to see my point of view."

Dentist: I guess if I were in your shoes, I'd be pretty upset too.

Comment: The dentist agrees that, from the patient's point of view, his angry feelings are understandable. Note that the dentist does not assume blame for the problem, he simply agrees that the patient's feelings are legitimate in the situation.

Patient: Well, what happened? How could decay start under the crown?

Comment: The patient is still upset, but he is no longer angry with the dentist. His question is probably a genuine request for information.

Dentist: If plaque and calculus build up around the crown, decay can start underneath.

Patient: Oh. (*Pause*) I guess I didn't realize that. I just assumed that the crown would protect any tooth left under it.

Dentist: I wish it were that simple.

Patient: So do I. (*Sighs*) Well, when do you want to remove the crown?

THE DEPRESSED PATIENT

Students occasionally ask, "Is there really a need for dentists to learn about depression? Depression is a psychiatric disorder, not a dental problem." The practicing dentist who is sensitive to the needs of his patients knows better. While he might not be aware of the incidence of depressive illness in the population, he knows that it is not uncommon to encounter patients who are mildly to moderately depressed in his practice.*

He is aware, too, that depressive illness can have significant effects on oral health. Patients who are listless and depressed may not be motivated for good oral hygiene practices. Deterioration in oral health habits can be a telling sign in a patient who has previously complied well with his recommendations for home care.

More importantly, however, depressive illness may influence oral health more directly through physiological changes which accompany both depression itself and the medications used to treat depression. Extensive research has shown that depressed patients have lower rates of salivary secretion than do normal control subjects.[7] This decreased rate of salivary secretion can alter the type and density of bacterial flora in the oral cavity, and

---

* *Despite major breakthroughs in the understanding and treatment of depression, depressive illness remains a health problem of considerable significance. It is estimated that a person's lifetime expectancy for developing a neurotic depression is about 20 to 30 percent—or between one chance in five and one in three.[5] Depression accounts for 75 percent of all psychiatric hospitalizations and, during any given year, 15 percent of all adults between the ages of 18 and 74 may suffer significant depressive symptoms.[6]*

several studies have reported an inverse relationship between rate of salivary flow and the incidence of carious lesions.[8,9]

The problem of salivary flow rate is compounded when the depressed patient is treated with tricyclic antidepressants, such as amitriptyline, imipramine, and doxepin. The anticholinergic action of this class of drugs is quite marked, especially during the early weeks of treatment. When these drugs are used in combination with phenothiazines or antiparkinsonian drugs, as is often the case, the problem of dry mouth occurs with even greater frequency.

The patient's vulnerability to caries is increased still further if, like many patients, he attempts to relieve the unpleasant sensation of dry mouth by sucking on hard candy, chewing gum, or sipping sweetened beverages. In one such case reported in the literature, a woman with a history of not more than two to three cavities per year developed 28 caries during a single depressive episode which was treated with a phenothiazine and a tricyclic antidepressant.[10]

The authors of this article suggest the use of fluoride lozenges for symptomatic relief of dry mouth. Although they also note that pilocarpine hydrochloride has been found useful in the treatment of dry mouth, they caution against side effects.

An additional note of caution is in order concerning depressed patients undergoing psychopharmacotherapy for depressive illness. As you are no doubt aware, administering solutions containing noradrenaline and solutions which contain 1:25,000 adrenaline should be avoided. Such solutions, in combination with tricyclic antidepressants or MAOI antidepressants, can produce severe headache, hypertension, and even death.[11]

Finally, it is important to be alert for signs of depression in patients who complain of chronic pain or pain for which no organic cause is apparent. Depression plays a significant role in pain perception and pain behavior. Studies show that over one-third of patients who appear in medical and dental clinics with primary complaints of pain are, in fact, depressed. Not infrequently, the "masked" or "hidden" depression is not detected until after several mechanical or surgical interventions have failed to produce lasting pain relief. The topic of pain is treated in detail in Chapter 5.

The Dentist's Role

How can you be of help to the depressed patient? The answer to this question depends on several factors, including the severity of the depression and whether or not the patient is already receiving treatment for his depressive illness.

The first step involves identification of the depressed patient. What cues signal the presence of depressive illness? The depressed patient often indicates his depressed state by his appearance and motor behavior. He may appear sad, listless, or "down in the dumps," although some depressed individuals appear irritable, anxious, and agitated.

Verbal behavior is often an important and obvious clue, but one which is overlooked with surprising frequency. Patients are sometimes quite willing to talk about how miserable they feel, but professionals, because of their own discomfort, are not always willing to listen. When a patient does express such feelings, avoid the temptation to "joke him out of it" or to provide false reassurance. A major symptom of depression is a pessimistic view of the future and a tendency to focus on and exaggerate current difficulties. Telling such a patient, "Everything will be all right" is of little comfort; he is quite sure that nothing will ever be all right again.

The patient who cries or appears on the verge of tears can be upsetting to the professional, who is likely to feel helpless and embarrassed. Often the professional may try to change the subject or provide reassurance and support in an effort to ward off tears. Yet, as Enlow and Swisher[12] point out, "fighting tears often results in the patient not being able to speak," while crying "often affords relief of severe depressive feelings and may make it possible for the patient to resume his account." These authors, who have made extensive studies of the doctor–patient relationship, add that an opportunity to cry may help the patient feel closer to the professional. They recommend not only that the patient be permitted to "cry it out," but that the clinician actually encourage or invite crying in a patient who appears on the verge of tears with a comment such as, "You look like you are about to cry."

Of course, we all have bad days—even bad weeks. How can you distinguish between a patient who is simply having a bad day and one who is truly, perhaps seriously, depressed? To help you decide, you will want to know the following:

- How long has the patient felt this way? Can he trace the onset of his current state to a specific precipitating event? It is sometimes mistakenly believed that, if a reason can be found to "explain" an episode of depression, the depression isn't a "real" depression. This is not the case, however, as true depressive episodes can follow sad or stressful life events.
- Has the patient's current mood and state interfered with his work or his usual routine? Have his interpersonal relationships been affected?

It is useful, too, to know if somatic symptoms are present. Sleep disturbances, including difficulty falling asleep, poor or restless sleep, and early morning awakening are very common in depressed patients. Gastrointestinal complaints are common, as is loss of appetite and weight. Menstrual changes in women and lowered sex drive and impaired sexual performance are also encountered.

If you have reason to believe that a patient is depressed, you will want to suggest that he seek appropriate help. You might say, for example:

> Mrs. Jones, I'm a little worried about you. You seem pretty low, pretty depressed. Do you think it might be helpful to see someone about this?

This questioning note leaves the door open for the patient to express her feelings about your suggestion. Many depressed patients are not aware that they are suffering from a depressive illness, as depression can manifest itself in many forms. Some, of course, might object to a referral to a psychiatrist or psychologist. For these patients, an acceptable alternative might be to see their family doctor, although this is a less than optimal solution. Patients are often more willing to consider seeking help if they are informed that depressive illness often responds quickly and dramatically to psychopharmacological intervention.

The dentist will rarely, if ever, be faced with a patient who is severely depressed, as such patients are typically too immobilized by their illness to present themselves for dental treatment. Similarly, it is probably rare for the dentist to encounter patients who are at immediate risk for suicide. If, however, you have any reason to believe that a patient might be at risk for suicide, obtain his permission to speak with his family. The patient should then be referred to a mental health professional (psychologist or psychiatrist) for immediate evaluation and treatment.

Because you will have occasion to make referrals to mental health professionals, it is a good idea to familiarize yourself with the resources in your area. If you do not know any mental health professionals, the community mental health center in your area is an appropriate starting point.

THE ANXIOUS PATIENT

Formal treatment methods to reduce excessive fear of dental treatment are presented in Chapter 4. In this section, we will confine our discussion to some general remarks concerning communication with the anxious patient. As it is probably the rare patient who does not experience at least an occasional twinge of anxiety in the dental operatory, this discussion applies to most of the patients you will encounter in your practice.

Communication with the anxious patient is complicated by the fact that dentists and patients tend to see dental events from very different viewpoints. Eric Jackson[13] offers an excellent example:

What is a root canal? To a dentist, a root canal is a small area of radiolucency around the apex of a tooth, which is going to go away because the tooth now has a smoothly reamed and filed radicular canal that has been beautifully and compactly filled. It is neat, tidy, clean, and will last for a long time. To the patient, (a root canal is) . . . a painful, horrifying, terrible last resort—like the thumbscrew.

Doctor Jackson's research reveals clear-cut differences between dentist and patient perceptions of dental events. His findings indicate that dentists and dental personnel acknowledge that patients are afraid of such high-stress events as injections and having a tooth removed, but that they fail to note patients' fear of what might be thought of as low-stress events, such as the dentist placing his fingertips in the patient's mouth and the dentist asking the patient to rinse his mouth. Such discrepancies in perception can, and probably often do, interfere with understanding and rapport between dentist and patient.

Communication with the anxious patient is further complicated by the fact that anxiety is not always simple to detect. While some highly anxious patients are easily recognized by their behavior, this is not always the case—especially if the patient attempts to conceal his fear from you. As we noted in a previous section, hostile behavior sometimes serves to mask underlying anxiety, and you must always be alert to the possibility that a touchy, defensive patient is really quite anxious beneath the disguise. When you respond to such patients in a nondefensive, reflective fashion, the patient's hostile behavior often diminishes. He may even be able to admit his apprehension, although this is not always the case.

Some patients may openly admit their feelings of apprehension but even these patients may be embarrassed by this admission. This is especially likely to be the case with male patients, as men are socialized to present a "manly front." Sensing such embarrassment in a patient, you might be reluctant to mention the patient's apparent discomfort. However, because attempts to conceal anxiety can actually lead to increased apprehension, the anxious patient may be difficult to work with until the anxiety itself has been discussed openly. A simple comment such as, "You seem a little tense," or "You look worried" is often enough to let the patient know that his feelings have been understood and accepted. Even if you have misjudged—if the patient is not, in fact, anxious—there is little harm done, as most patients will appreciate your concern and your attempts to understand.

Many dentists make the mistake of telling an anxious patient to relax, much as they might instruct him to open his mouth or turn slightly to one side. This is like telling someone not to think about pink elephants—a suggestion which inevitably produces results opposite from those desired. It should be obvious that patients do not choose to remain tense and anxious and that, if relaxation were under voluntary control, they would relax without the need to be told. It is even more confusing to tell a patient to "try to relax." This is tantamount to instructing him to make an effort to relax. In most cases, the harder the patient tries to relax the more tense he will become, as he finds himself unable to comply with the dentist's instructions.

Fear of the unknown is one of the most powerful factors in producing anxiety in any situation, in the dental setting or elsewhere. No matter how minor and routine a procedure seems to you, it may be viewed as major, complex, and frightening by the patient. Most dentists are aware of this and are careful to provide thorough explanations of procedures prior to initiating them. However, because anxiety interferes with the ability to listen and comprehend, you should always check to be sure the patient understands exactly what will be done, the length of time involved, and what sensations he can expect to experience.

Most dentists probably agree on the importance of avoiding frightening or threatening words when explaining procedures or describing sensations. One dentist[14] who has written on the subject of semantics (the study of human response to symbols and symbol systems, including language) suggests that the following words be avoided: cut, drill, scrape, chisel, knife, scale, needle, pliers, and cement. He recommends the following phrases and terms:

Prepare a tooth		Grind down a tooth
Remove a tooth		Pull a tooth
Restore a tooth	*instead of*	Fill a tooth
Dentures		Plates
Smooth		File
Investment		Cost

The dentist's verbal behavior is important throughout the dental visit. During treatment, encouraging remarks such as "Very nice," "Good," and "This is going to feel a lot more comfortable" let the patient know that you are aware that there is a person on the other end of the tooth. Especially during lengthy procedures, it is also a good idea to let the patient know that there is an end in sight. Comments such as "Not much longer now," and "I just have to do such-and-such, then we'll be finished," help relieve the patient's nagging suspicion that he will die of old age before the end of the appointment.

One final but important note concerning verbal behavior: criticism, when used at all, should be used with special caution with the anxious patient. Although dentists sometimes employ criticism as a means of motivating patients to improve their oral health practices, this tactic can boomerang and, in extreme cases, actually contribute to dental fear and avoidance. In fact, one researcher[15] reported that the most common cause of patient anxiety was "lest the dentist should adopt a negative attitude because of neglect of the teeth." In another study,[16] in which fearful and nonfearful patients ranked 25 fears associated with the dental situation, the item "Dentist tells you that you have bad teeth" was ranked third. Ranked seventh was "Dentist laughs as he looks in your mouth."

These studies underscore the importance to the patient of the dentist's attitude. They should serve to remind us that what we say to a patient is at least as important as what we do technically—in some cases, perhaps, even more important.

REFERENCES

1. Gamsky, N. R. and Farwell, G. F. "Counselor verbal behavior as a function of client hostility." *J Counsl Psychol* 13:184, 1966.
2. Ingersoll, B. D. and Tetkoski, M. "Dentist-patient communication: What do patients want to hear?" Unpublished manuscript, West Virginia University School of Dentistry, 1980.
3. Bernstein, L.; Bernstein, R. S.; Dana, R. H. *Interviewing: A Guide for Health Professionals.* New York: Appleton-Century-Crofts, 1974.
4. Singer, J. "Avoiding patient relation stress in an orthodontic practice." *Am J Orthodont* 75:173, 1979.
5. Klerman, G. "Affective disorders." In *The Harvard Guide to Modern Psychiatry*, edited by A. Nicholi. Cambridge, Mass.: Harvard University Press, Belknap Press, 1978.
6. Secunda, S. K.; Katz, M. M.; Friedman, R. J.; Schuyler, D. "Special Report: 1973—The Depressive Disorders." Washington, D.C.: Government Printing Office, 1973.
7. Gottlieb, G. and Paulson, G. "Salivation in depressed patients." *Arch Gen Psychiat* 5:468, 1961.
8. Hyde, E. J. "Salivary flow rate of children and its relationship to dental caries." *Canad Dent A J* 5:186, 1972.
9. Ericson, T.; Nordblom, A.; Ekedahl, C. "Effects on caries suceptibility after surgical treatment of drooling in patients with neurological disorders." *Acta Otolaryn* 75:71, 1973.
10. Bassuk, E. and Schoonover, S. "Rampant dental caries in the treatment of depression." *J Clin Psychiat* 39(2):163, 1978.
11. Hordern, A. "Dental dilemmas: Can psychiatry help?" *Austral Dent J* 22:295, 1977.
12. Enlow, A. J. and Swisher, S. N. *Interviewing and Patient Care.* 2d ed. New York: Oxford University Press, 1979.
13. Jackson, E: "Patients' perceptions of dentistry." In *Advances in Behavioral Research*

in Dentistry, edited by P. Weinstein. Seattle: University of Washington, 1978.
14. Jan, H. "General semantic orientation in dentist-patient relations." *Am Dent A J* 68:424, 1964.
15. Forsberg, A. "Odontologiska fakulteten vid Karolinska institutet, Tandnards-sbraeb." *Seven Tandlak Tidskr* 59:147, 1966.
16. Gale, E. "Fears of the dental situation." *J Dent Res* 51:964, 1972.

4

The Origins and Treatment of Dental Fear

The fearful dental patient is a popular subject of humor in jokes and cartoons, but to a sizeable number of people in the general population, fear of dental treatment is no laughing matter. While most people would probably admit to occasional feelings of mild apprehension concerning dental treatment, many people experience such intense fear that they simply avoid going to the dentist. Surveys show that the number of people so affected may be as high as five to six percent of the population, or 11 to 13 million people.[1,2] As a group, women report more fear of dentistry than men,[3] and children report more fear than adults.

Fear of dental treatment is a problem not only for the fearful patient but for his dentist as well. Anxious patients often require more time per visit, even for simple procedures. In addition, working with tense, anxious patients can be a source of considerable stress for all members of the dental team. Fear is the patient problem most frequently cited by dentists, and it ranks among patient problems dentists consider most serious or important.[4]

Younger dentists (those in practice for less than ten years) identify this problem as particularly common.[4] This may be because they have not yet learned how to put patients at ease, or it may be because they simply have not had enough contact, over time, with their patients to establish relationships characterized by mutual trust and respect. Such a relationship, as we have discussed, can help reduce patient anxiety and apprehension.

Endodontists and periodontists also report encountering fearful patients with great frequency.[4] Again, these specialists may have insufficient contact with a patient to enable the patient to overcome his fear. In addition, the average patient knows little about endodontic and periodontic procedures and may perceive them as especially frightening—even terrifying.

Fear is an important factor in missed or cancelled appointments. It is not surprising that fearful patients are far more likely to fail appointments than less fearful patients. In fact, one investigator reported the incidence of missed appointments as three times greater among high-fear patients than among low-fear patients.[5]

In this chapter, we will focus on the origins, assessment, and treatment of dental fear in adult patients.

ORIGINS AND DEVELOPMENT OF DENTAL FEAR

Is dental fear associated with certain traits or a specific "type" of personality? Is fear of dentistry a symptom of underlying unconscious conflict? Early studies of dental fear sought to answer these questions. However, attempts to uncover the origins of dental fear within the patient's unconscious and to identify personality characteristics associated with fear of dentistry were not successful. Researchers so far have failed to find relationships between dental fear and such personality traits as orality, dependency, trouble with authority figures, neuroticism, or introversion–extroversion.[6,7]

However, these studies did reveal significant differences between fearful and nonfearful patients in reported dental history and in family attitudes toward dentistry. Specifically, fearful patients more frequently reported a history of traumatic dental experiences and unfavorable family attitudes toward dentistry.

Traumatic Experiences

Psychologists Ronald Kleinknecht and Douglas Bernstein have conducted a major series of investigations into the origins, assessment, and treatment of dental fear. Their work has provided additional support for the role of traumatic dental experiences in the development of dental fear. These authors[8] surveyed 225 college students, 93 of whom were highly fearful of dentistry and 132 who were not fearful. These students were asked to describe specific experiences with dentistry which they considered instrumental in forming their present attitudes. Responses were then classified as "positive" or "negative." An example of a positive response is the statement:

> My dentist was patient and gentle and seemed to make a sincere effort to avoid unnecessary pain. He had me signal him with my hand when it hurt, then he would wait until I was OK before proceeding.

An example of a negative response is the statement:

> My dentist bugged me a lot. He would become angry if I felt pain.
> He pushed my hair around and lectured constantly about young
> people and their hair.

Of the total responses given by the high-fear students, almost three-quarters (71 percent) were classified as negative, while less than half (47 percent) of the responses given by low-fear students were negative. Note, however, that the high-fear group did make some positive comments, just as the low-fear group made some negative comments.

Table 4-1 shows the proportion within each group describing a specific aspect of dentistry as negative. You can see, for example, that about half of the high-fear students made negative comments about the dentist's behavior and personality, while less than a third of the low-fear group made such comments. Similarly, among high-fear students, 42 percent complained of painful experiences, compared with only 17 percent of the low-fear students.

Kleinknecht was careful to point out that pain itself cannot be explained as the cause of fear, as 17 percent of the low-fear group reported painful experiences yet did not develop fear. Further, 81 percent of those in the high-fear group who reported negatively on dentist behavior did not cite pain. Kleinknecht hypothesized that, "It may well be that it is not pain itself but rather how the dentist deals with the patient who experiences pain that causes fear."[8]

Influence of Friends and Family

Throughout their lives, human beings learn from observing the behavior of others. Initially, it is the family, the child's earliest source of information about his world, which exerts the strongest influence on the development of

TABLE 4-1. PERCENT OF EACH GROUP CITING SPECIFIC ASPECTS OF DENTISTRY AS NEGATIVE.

	High-fear Students	Low-fear Students
Dentist's behavior and personality	51	30
Pain	42	17
Anesthetic injection	35	12

Kleinknecht, R. A. "Fear and avoidance of dentistry." In P. Weinstein (ed): *Advances in Behavioral Research in Dentistry*. Seattle: University of Washington Press, 1978.

an individual's attitudes, beliefs, and behavior. As the child grows, the peer group gradually replaces the family as the primary source of influence, and friends become an increasingly important factor in shaping attitudes and behavior.

Results of recent studies have supported the findings of earlier research. We know that family attitudes are an important factor in the development of dental fear. In one recent study,[3] a survey was administered to several hundred students who ranged in age from junior high school to graduate school. These students were asked to describe what they thought were important factors in determining their present attitudes toward dentistry. The most commonly offered reason for negative attitudes was negative expectations learned from others. Almost one-fifth (17 percent) of the respondents stated that information from family and friends led them to expect unpleasant experiences in the dental operatory. Other studies have shown that the parents of very fearful children were themselves dentally fearful as children and that they remain anxious as adults.

Childhood friends and siblings are an especially frequent source of negative expectations. This finding is consistent with the results of another study in which fourth-grade children, asked to list sources of positive and negative information about dentistry, cited friends and siblings more frequently than any other group as sources of negative information.[9]

THE ASSESSMENT OF DENTAL FEAR

Accurate detection and assessment of dental fear is important for both clinical and research purposes. If you are to take precautionary measures or use special procedures when treating fearful patients, you must first be able to identify these patients. Further, you must be able to distinguish between patients who are only slightly fearful and those whose fear is intense, as management strategies for each may differ.

The researcher, too, must be able to assess levels of fear. Otherwise, he could not undertake investigations which involve separating subjects into high-fear and low-fear groups to examine differences between the groups. In addition, without accurate methods of assessment, we could not evaluate the effectiveness of various treatments designed to reduce or eliminate dental fear.

Fear is a complex phenomenon. Any definition of fear must, of course, include the individual's report of subjectively experienced discomfort or apprehension. The subjective feeling of fear is also accompanied by physiological changes, such as increased heart rate and increased sweat gland activity. Often, too, we see changes in overt behavior, such as crying, trembling, or running away.

Activity occurring in each of these channels can be measured, and these measures can be used to indicate level of fear. In the assessment of dental fear, research measures which have been used singly and in combination include self-report measures, physiological measures, and observation of overt behavior. While only a few of these measures are suitable for routine office use, a variety are included in our discussion, both to dispel some common myths and because you will encounter them in your reading of the dental literature.

Self-Report Measures

Perhaps the most straightforward way to determine whether a person feels fearful is to ask him. Researchers have devised a variety of questionnaires for this purpose, but before a questionnaire can be considered useful, it must be shown to produce scores which are both valid and reliable. Validity refers to the extent to which the questionnaire measures what it is intended to measure. In the case of dental fear, validity is usually established by demonstrating that scores on the questionnaire correlate with scores on other measures of fear, such as overt behavior or changes in heart rate or sweat gland activity.

Reliability concerns the consistency of scores or the likelihood that subjects will obtain the same or similar scores if the questionnaire is administered on several occasions. Scientists use statistical procedures to determine the reliability of a measuring device.

Several questionnaires have been developed to assess dental fear. Two of the most commonly used are the Dental Anxiety Scale[10] and the Dental Fear Survey.[3] Both have been shown to be valid and reliable measures of dental fear.

The Dental Anxiety Scale, reproduced in Figure 4-1, is a four-item questionnaire which can be used in the dental office or in research projects. The scale, which takes the patient only a few minutes to complete, yields a single summary score. The authors state that a score of 13 or 14 "should make the dentist suspicious that he is dealing with an anxious patient." They add that patients who earn a score of 15 or more are almost always highly anxious.[11]

The Dental Fear Survey, reproduced in Figure 4-2, is a longer questionnaire which also yields a summary score. (In this case, the individual's score on Item 20 is considered the summary score. The authors consider a score of one or two to indicate low fear, a score of four or five high fear.) In addition, this questionnaire also provides information about the patient's responses to specific stimuli associated with the dental experience, such as the smell of the operatory and the sight of the instruments.

Using this questionnaire, these authors found that the sight of the syringe; the sensation of the anesthetic injection; and the sight, sound, and sen-

1. If you had to go to the dentist tommorrow, how would you feel about it?
   a. I would look forward to it as a reasonably enjoyable experience
   b. I wouldn't care one way or the other
   c. I would be a little uneasy about it
   d. I would be afraid that it would be unpleasant and painful
   e. I would be very frightened of what the dentist might do
2. When you are waiting in the dentist's office for your turn in the chair, how do you feel?
   a. Relaxed
   b. A little uneasy
   c. Tense
   d. Anxious
   e. So anxious that I sometimes break out in a sweat or almost feel physically sick
3. When you are in the dentist's chair waiting while he gets his drill ready to begin working on your teeth, how do you feel?
   a. Relaxed
   b. A little uneasy
   c. Tense
   d. Anxious
   e. So anxious that I sometimes break out in a sweat or almost feel physically sick
4. You are in the dentist's chair to have your teeth cleaned. While you are waiting and the dentist is getting out the instruments which he will use to scrape your teeth around the gums, how do you feel?
   a. Relaxed
   b. A little uneasy
   c. Tense
   d. Anxious
   e. So anxious that I sometimes break out in a sweat or almost feel physically sick

FIG. 4-1. Dental Anxiety Scale. *Corah, N. L. "Development of a dental anxiety scale." Journal of Dental Research 48:596, 1969. Reprinted by permission.*

sation of the drill produced the highest fear ratings among their respondents. The authors cautioned that "few patients are typical and each will have a particular pattern of fear responses within the dental treatment situation." While this is almost certainly true, the findings from this study nevertheless provide valuable guidelines as to the most common fear stimuli and serve to focus the attention of clinician and researcher upon them.*

---

* *Interestingly, in a later study, these authors found that the nature of the specific treatment procedures performed during the appointment did not relate to fear expressed. Patients found bridgework, crowns, and root canals no more stressful than amalgam restorations.*[5]

Please rate your feeling or reaction on these items using the following scale:

1	**2**	**3**	**4**	**5**
never	once or twice	a few times	often	nearly everytime

_____ 1. Has fear of dental work ever caused you to put off making an appointment?

_____ 2. Has fear of dental work ever caused you to cancel or not appear for an appointment?

When having dental work done: (use the following scale)

1	**2**	**3**	**4**	**5**
not at all	a little	somewhat	much	very much

_____ 3. My muscles become tense

_____ 4. My breathing rate increases

_____ 5. I perspire

_____ 6. I feel nauseated and sick to my stomach

_____ 7. My heart beats faster

Using the scale above, please rate how much fear, anxiety, or unpleasantness each of the following causes you.

_____ 8. Making an appointment for dentistry

_____ 9. Approaching the dentist's office

_____ 10. Sitting in the waiting room

_____ 11. Being seated in the dental operatory

_____ 12. The smell of the dentist's office

_____ 13. Seeing the dentist walk in

_____ 14. Seeing the anesthetic needle

_____ 15. Feeling the needle injected

_____ 16. Seeing the drill

_____ 17. Hearing the drill

_____ 18. Feeling the vibrations of the drill

_____ 19. Having your teeth cleaned

_____ 20. All things considered, how fearful are you of having dental work done?

FIG. 4-2. Dental Fear Survey. *Kleinknecht, R. A.; Klepac, R. K.; Alexander, L. D. "Origins and characteristics of fear of dentistry." American Dental Association Journal 86:842, 1973. Reprinted by permission.*

Physiological Measures

Changes in activity within the autonomic nervous system often accompany self-reports of fear. These changes include increases in cardiac rate, peripheral blood flow, and sweat gland activity as well as changes in gastric activity, respiration, and pupillary responding.

The physiological measures most commonly used in studies of dental fear are changes in palmar sweat gland activity and changes in the electrical activity of the skin. A measure of palmar sweat gland activity is the Palmar Sweat Index (PSI), obtained by applying a graphite solution to the finger. When this substance dries, it is peeled off and mounted on a slide for microscopic examination. Open sweat pores, which appear as holes in the film, are counted and the total employed as a measure of sweat gland activity. Using this measure, Kleinknecht and Bernstein[14] found that low-fear subjects adapted to the dental situation over the course of the dental appointment, as indicated by decreases in PSI scores across the appointment. Such a pattern of steady decline was not found among high-fear subjects, suggesting that these subjects do not adapt during the appointment.

Electrodes attached to the fingers with paste are used to monitor changes in the electrical activity of the skin. The researcher can measure changes in galvanic skin resistance (GSR) or its converse, galvanic skin conductance (GSC). The frequency with which such changes occur is used as an indicator of arousal or fear. For example, the anesthetic injection is associated with greatest frequency of change in GSR, followed by high-speed drilling, then by low-speed drilling.[12]

Increases in cardiac rate are also associated with feelings of fear. Significant differences have been found between the cardiac rate scores of fearful children and those of nonfearful children during dental treatment, with fearful children showing higher mean cardiac rate.[13] Similar findings have been reported with adult patients.[11]

Measures of Overt Behavior

In the study of dental fear, one important category of behavior is cancelling or missing appointments. As previously noted, fearful patients miss or cancel appointments far more frequently than nonfearful patients. Other behaviors of interest include body movements and speech in the reception area and the operatory.

If asked, "Who moves about more during dental treatment, fearful patients or nonfearful patients?" most people would probably respond, "Fearful patients." In the popular imagination, the fearful patient is one who taps his feet, drums his fingers, and talks a great deal to hold the dentist at bay. We might also expect to see trembling and gripping of the chair arms and to hear grunts, squeals, and requests for the dentist to stop.

Surprisingly, this does not seem to be the case. In the dental operatory, fearful adult patients not only do not move around or verbalize more than nonfearful patients, in some cases they may even exhibit less movement.[15] In studies comparing the behavior of low-fear patients with that of high-fear patients, Kleinknecht and Bernstein[14] recorded the reception area and operatory behavior of each subject on videotape. The videotapes were coded by trained observers who recorded general activities (such as talking or reading), specific activities (such as hand, foot, arm, and head movements), and posture (such as grips chair arm, crosses legs).

Differences between the groups were found only in waiting room behavior. In the reception area, high-fear subjects moved their arms more and engaged in more movements and/or activities than low-fear subjects. In the operatory, there were no differences between the groups.

The failure to find differences in gross body movements or verbalizations between two groups of adult patients probably reflects the fact that adult behavior is typically under strong control of social cues. Most adults are aware that it is inappropriate to thrash about and scream during dental treatment and this awareness functions to inhibit such behavior.

This notion is supported by the finding that, when asked about details of the assessment appointment several months after the appointment, many patients—especially those in the high-fear group—recalled engaging in much more movement than was actually observed.[8] Further, they recalled doing things which were seldom or never observed, such as yawning, stretching, or jumping. We can guess that patients may think about or feel like engaging in these behaviors but that they are prevented by social demands of the situation.

It may be, of course, that more subtle body movements can be identified that will distinguish between fearful and nonfearful adult patients. However, it is clear from the evidence to date that the dentist who relies only on overt behavior as an indicator of patient anxiety is very likely to be in error concerning his assessment.

REDUCING DENTAL FEAR

Because even the nonfearful patient can become sensitized and fearful of dental treatment if he is mismanaged, it is important that dentists know and follow certain guidelines relative to fear with all patients, not just those who describe themselves as very fearful. Dr. Eric Jackson, a dentist who has also been trained as a psychologist, suggests the following rules that dentists might find useful on a day to day basis.[16]

1. *Do not inflict pain if it is possible to avoid doing so.* Although this rule may seem too obvious to mention, Dr. Jackson rightly points out that pain can sensitize a previously nonfearful patient. He urges that dentists use "all means" at their disposal to eliminate pain.

2. *Accidental pain should cease immediately.* Avoid the temptation to finish the job without stopping. Use additional anesthetic, or if that is not possible, stop work and warn the patient of additional impending discomfort before proceeding.
3. *If there is any possibility that the patient will feel pain, warn him.* Unpredictable aversive events are much more stressful than aversive events which are predictable. An accurate description of impending painful events helps the patient prepare for the event and enables him to cope more effectively with it.
4. *Other than the situation described in Rule 3, avoid using emotion-charged words like "pain" and "hurt."* Substitute less threatening words such as "discomfort" and "tenderness."
5. *If you say, "This will not be uncomfortable," be absolutely sure you are correct.* This rule is the reciprocal of Rule 3. The patient cannot relax and trust you if he cannot believe what you say.
6. *Tell the patient that he can signal you to stop work by raising his hand. If he signals, stop immediately.* Control, like predictability, reduces the stress associated with aversive events. Few patients will actually need to make use of the signal; even fewer will abuse it.
7. *Introduce new procedures slowly and gently.* This extends even to entering the operatory. Dr. Jackson suggests that, with fearful patients, the dentist should remove his white coat and talk with the patient in the business office before entering the operatory.
8. *Praise desirable behaviors but never chastise for undesirable behaviors.* Many patients worry that the dentist will criticize them for poor oral hygiene and infrequent visits in the past. In fact, some even avoid dental treatment for this reason. As Dr. Jackson points out, even if the patient has been careless in the past, he is now seeking dental treatment and should be praised for doing so.
9. *The dental environment should be as quiet and relaxed as possible.* According to Dr. Jackson, a frantic, noisy environment increases a patient's general arousal level and potentiates fear. Remember to move and talk slowly and train your auxiliaries to do the same.

Treatment Methods for Dental Fear

Dental practitioners and students sometimes ask whether, in light of pharmocologic methods currently available, there is need for psychological methods for treating the fearful patient. On this question, we are in strong agreement with Gerald Wright's statement, "Drugs are not substitutes for the fundamental nonpharmacotherapeutic approaches to behavior management."[17]

With recent increased awareness of the possible harmful effects on the human body of insecticides, food additives, industrial pollutants, and other chemicals, patients and health care professionals alike have adopted a more conservative stance toward medication. Certainly, reports of unpleasant and even tragic long-range effects of some medications have reinforced this conservative trend, and it is not uncommon to encounter patients who are reluctant to take medication or drugs except for serious illness.

In addition, some patients cannot take medication due to allergies, other medical conditions, or possible adverse effects resulting from interaction with other medication. These patients obviously require nonpharmacologic management, as do patients whose intense fear prevents them from even appearing in a dental office.

If we were to judge from the number of articles in the dental literature describing psychological techniques for managing fear patients, we might reasonably conclude that few problems remain to be solved in this area. Unfortunately, however, most of the published articles are no more than anecdotal reports and subjective impressions based on personal experience. Certainly, this information can provide useful clinical leads, but it cannot help us decide on the relative merits of one treatment compared to others, nor can it tell us what success rate we can expect or what types of patients are most likely to benefit. This information can only be provided by careful research and controlled investigations. Such studies are being undertaken in several dental schools and psychology departments across the country. Although the data are only preliminary at this point, these studies provide promising leads for efficient and effective treatment of dental fear.

It is sometimes difficult to make clear distinctions between methods to reduce fear and those to reduce pain, as anxiety and pain are so often intertwined. Many believe that hypnosis, for example, brings about pain reduction by reducing associated anxiety. In this section, we will discuss treatments which are oriented primarily toward helping individuals overcome excessive fear. Methods designed primarily to reduce pain and bodily discomfort are discussed in the chapter dealing with pain.

Biofeedback Methods We have described a variety of physiological changes which accompany anxiety. Dental patients themselves describe muscle tension as the most commonly experienced physiological reaction to dental treatment, followed by salivation and by increases in heart rate, perspiration, and respiration.

These reports indicate that bodily changes during emotion, when they occur, do not go unnoticed by dental patients—especially very fearful patients. In fact, awareness of increased physiological arousal appears to play an important role in determining how an individual cognitively appraises his emotional state and the emotion-provoking situation. That is, if a patient undergoing dental treatment notices that his palms are moist and his heart is racing, he is likely to interpret these changes as an indication that he is, indeed, quite upset and will probably label the situation as more frightening and himself as more frightened than might have been the case otherwise. In such a way, a feedback loop is set up and awareness of increased physiological arousal can lead to further increases in anxiety.

If perceived increases in physiological arousal can lead to increased anxiety, might the reverse also be true? By reducing levels of physiological arousal, can we produce concomitant decreases in subjectively experienced anxiety and discomfort? This, of course, is the rationale underlying biofeedback, an approach which is aimed at helping patients learn to control their levels of physiological arousal. Biofeedback procedures involve measuring physiological activity, transforming this information into a signal such as a light or a tone, and training the patient to use this signal to alter the level of physiological activity.

In his laboratory, dentist-psychologist Richard Hirschman has investigated the effectiveness of various biofeedback procedures as a means of reducing stress during dental treatment. Using electromyographic (EMG) feedback, Dr. Hirschman[18] trained dental patients to decrease muscle activity in the forearm, a training procedure which can be accomplished in a single, brief session. Highly anxious patients who received biofeedback were less anxious during treatment and experienced the restorative procedures as less stressful than they had anticipated. In contrast, highly anxious patients in the no-treatment control group showed *increases* in anxiety and experienced the restorative procedures as *more* stressful than anticipated.

Dr. Hirschman and his research group have also studied the effects of a simple procedure known as "paced respiration." Their studies[19] indicate that, when highly anxious patients use a signal light to pace their respiration at a slower-than-normal rate, they rate dental treatment as less unpleasant than patients who breathe at a normal or faster-than-normal rate.

Promising results, too, have been obtained with heart-rate feedback.[19] In an interesting series of studies, subjects who received inaccurate feedback (indicating decreases in heart rate when increases were actually occurring, or increases when heart rate was really decreasing) responded like subjects who received accurate feedback. Regardless of the accuracy of the feedback, subjects who received feedback indicating heart rate decreases rated dental stimuli as less unpleasant than those who were given feedback indicating increases in heart rate. These results are significant, as they suggest that actual magnitude or direction of visceral change—or even whether change occurs at all—might not be particularly important: as long as the patient believes that decreases in his own physiological activity are taking place, he is likely to label himself as more comfortable and relaxed.

Whatever the mechanism by which these results are produced, the evidence indicates that biofeedback procedures offer promise in the dental operatory, especially with highly anxious patients. The procedures themselves are efficient and relatively brief and can be implemented by a dental auxiliary. Equipment requirements are modest and reliable instruments can be obtained at reasonable cost.

A good overview for the clinician interested in biofeedback is *Biofeedback: Principles and Practice for Clinicians.** An additional source of information is: The Biofeedback Society of America, 4301 Owens Street, Wheat Ridge, Colorado 80033.

Relaxation and Systematic Desensitization The method of treating excessive fear now known as "systematic desensitization" has a long history. In 1924, Mary Cover Jones successfully desensitized a young child who was intensely afraid of rabbits by gradually moving the rabbit closer to the child while the child was engaged in eating his favorite food.

This technique of substituting a nonfearful response for a fearful response was futher explored by Joseph Wolpe, who worked initially with laboratory animals taught to fear a cage in which they had received electric shock. When placed in the shock cage, the animals continued to show intense fear, even when shock was no longer presented. In other, dissimilar cages, the animals showed less fear. By moving the animals through a series of cages, each more like the shock cage than the previous cage, and by feeding them in each cage, Wolpe was able to eliminate fear of the shock cage.

Wolpe then extended his work to the study of fearful human subjects.[20] However, instead of feeding his human subjects, Wolpe used a simplified version of progressive relaxation training, a method which employs alternate tensing and relaxing of various muscle groups in the body (see Appendix A).

A hierarchy of anxiety-producing situations was constructed for each individual, specific to his particular fear. For a patient who fears dogs, for example, the lowest item in the hierarchy might be, "looking at pictures of dogs in a book." The highest item in this person's hierarchy might be, "petting a large German Shepard" or "walking past a yard in which a big dog is growling menacingly."

The patient was taught to relax and instructed to visualize a scene from the low fear end of his hierarchy. Gradually, while in a relaxed state, the patient progressed through all items in his hierarchy, just as the laboratory animals progressed through a series of cages before finally reaching the shock cage.

Eventually, patients were able to remain relaxed while visualizing the most frightening situations in their hierarchies. Generalization to the real situation occurred, so that the patients were able to remain calm when ac-

---

* *Basmajian, J. V. (ed), Baltimore; Williams and Wilkins Co., 1979.*

tually confronted with situations which previously had been very frightening to them.

Wolpe's method has been applied successfully to a very broad range of irrational fears. Among the fears successfully treated are fear of animals, snakes, insects, injections, water, crowds, and flying, to name only a few.

The first report of successful treatment of dental fear using systematic desensitization was published by Gale and Ayer in 1969.[21] These authors described the case of a 32-year-old man who reported intense fear of dental treatment since childhood. So intense was his fear that he could not obtain dental treatment necessary to enlist in the Marine Corps, nor could he obtain treatment for repeated painful toothaches. Treatment consisted of nine one-hour sessions during which the patient was trained in relaxation, the hierarchy was constructed (see Fig. 4-3), and hierarchy items were presented while the patient was relaxed. Just prior to the ninth desensitization session, the patient made and kept a dental appointment. After the ninth session, the patient attended three additional dental appointments and completed all necessary dental treatment, including restorations and extractions. The authors added that patient now describes dental treatment as "relaxing."

Other case reports have also suggested that systematic desensitization can be an effective means of reducing dental fear. In an interesting study conducted by Dr. Robert Klepac,[22] three of five dental avoiders who were

---

1. Thinking about going to the dentist
2. Getting in your car to go to the dentist
3. Calling for an appointment with the dentist
4. Sitting in the waiting room of the dentist's office
5. Having the nurse tell you it's your turn
6. Getting in the dentist's chair
7a. Seeing the dentist lay out his instruments, one of which is a probe
7b. Seeing the dentist lay out his instruments, one of which is pliers that are used to pull teeth
8. Having a probe held in front of you while you look at it
9. Having a probe placed on the side of a tooth
10. Having a probe placed in a cavity
11. Getting an injection in your gums on one side
12a. Having your teeth drilled and worrying that the anesthetic will wear off
12b. Having a tooth pulled
13a. Getting an injection on each side
13b. Hearing the crunching sounds as your tooth is being pulled

---

FIG. 4-3. Patient's hierarchy. *Gale, E. N. and Ayer, W. A. "Treatment of dental phobias." American Dental Association Journal 78:1304, 1969. Reprinted with permission.*

treated with systematic desensitization were then able to complete a course of dental treatment. For two patients, however, it was necessary to use additional procedures before they successfully completed dental treatment.

In a controlled investigation,[23] nine long-term dental avoiders were treated with systematic desensitization. At follow-up three months after treatment, four patients had completed all or almost all necessary dental work, two had obtained emergency treatment, and three had not visited a dentist at all.

The results of these studies suggest that systematic desensitization is an effective method of reducing dental fear in some patients. However, success rates with fearful dental patients are lower than those obtained for other types of fears. This is not surprising, as fear of dentistry differs in one very important respect from other "irrational" fears: even with modern treatment techniques and anesthetics, the dental patient can realistically expect to experience some degree of discomfort. In fact, the two patients in Klepac's study who required additional treatment cited pain as the reason for their continued fear.

Finally, we must point out that, although systematic desensitization is brief in comparison with more traditional, "in-depth" methods for treating fear, it is nevertheless a time-consuming procedure. Few dentists are in partnership with a psychologist and fewer still could be expected to find the time to provide this treatment themselves.

One means of reducing demands on costly professional time is to automate desensitization procedures. Promising results have resulted from allowing patients to view hierarchically presented scenes on videotape. Using this method with very fearful patients, one group of investigators reported that two-thirds of these patients subsequently made and kept dental treatment appointments.[24]

A less costly alternative is to provide the patient with audiotape cassettes containing relaxation instructions and scenes from a standard dental fear hierarchy.* The tapes and instructions for their use could be given to the patient at the initial examination or the prophylaxis visit, and the patient could listen to the tapes at home, repeating them as often as necessary.

Another low-cost alternative is simply to have the patient listen through headphones to a tape recording of relaxation instructions throughout the treatment appointment. In one study[25] in which patients were provided with such a tape at each of two restorative appointments, those who heard the relaxation tape showed significant reductions in self-reported discomfort and were rated as less anxious by the dentist. The effects of listening to the tape were especially beneficial to high-fear patients.

Both of these methods—relaxation tapes for office use and systematic desensitization tapes for home use—have the advantage of being low in cost

---

* See Appendix A for relaxation instructions and a sample hierarchy.

and simple to administer. Other promising alternatives are described in the following section.

Modeling We have seen that people can learn negative or fearful attitudes by listening to and observing others. It is reasonable to ask whether people can also learn new, more adaptive attitudes through the same observational process. An increasing amount of evidence indicates quite clearly that they can.

Albert Bandura, a psychologist at Stanford University, pioneered this approach in a major research program in which "models" were used to help fearful children and adults overcome various fears. Working initially with children, Bandura found that children who intensely feared and avoided dogs could be helped to overcome their fear by watching other children (models) interact fearlessly with dogs. A graduated approach similar to that used in systematic desensitization was used, so that the models progressed from less threatening situations, such as petting a dog through the bars of a cage, to situations which included very close contact with unconfined dogs.

Modeling has been extensively applied in the treatment of fearful, disruptive child patients. In addition to a number of case reports, several well-controlled studies have shown that, in general, children who view a cooperative child undergoing dental treatment are much less anxious and disruptive than children who do not observe such models or than children who are exposed to the commonly employed "Tell-Show-Do" approach.[26,27] It may be that models provide a child not only with information about what to expect in the dental situation but also about how to behave in that situation.

The opportunity to observe models undergoing dental treatment is also a useful method for reducing fear in adult dental patients, as a number of studies have shown. Success rates reported for the use of this method with fearful, avoidant patients are about 55–60 percent.[24]

It is not necessary to have a live model present in order to use a modeling approach. Filmed modeling has been shown to be as effective as the use of live models. The use of films or videotapes would not present major difficulties in the dental office, and filmed or taped material can be reviewed by the patient as often as necessary.

The dentist who is interested in using modeling to reduce dental fear should keep the following points in mind in designing a modeling treatment program:

- The observer (patient) is more likely to imitate the model's behavior if he observes the model receiving praise for his behavior (with children, trinkets or prizes can be given).
- The observer should view more than one model. As each model will vary slightly in the details of his behavior, the observer is exposed to a broader

range of specific adaptive behaviors by observing multiple models. Modeling effects are also enhanced if the observer perceives some similarity between himself and the model and, when multiple models are shown, where there is a greater likelihood that the observer will perceive at least a few models as being similiar to himself.

- It is particularly important that the observer perceive the model as similar to himself in fearfulness. Better results are obtained with models who initially appear somewhat timid and who are shown gradually overcoming their fear than with models who appear fearless and confident from the start.

Combined Procedures In general, modeling and desensitization procedures appear roughly comparable in effectiveness. Studies show that, using either method alone, success rates are about 55–60 percent* (that is, the method is effective in enabling about 55–60 percent of patients so treated to subsequently seek and receive dental treatment).

Much better results have been obtained by employing a combination of both methods in one treatment package. In two controlled studies,[22,27] dental avoiders were taught progressive relaxation and were then shown modeling films while relaxed. In both studies, success rates of 78 percent were obtained.

It may be of additional benefit if, following treatment with this combined approach, the patient is then permitted to spend some time becoming habituated to the dental setting before he actually undergoes dental treatment. Kleinknecht and Bernstein[29] followed this procedure with two dental avoiders, allowing each to spend 30 minutes in the waiting room and 30 minutes in the operatory with a dental assistant present to answer questions. Both patients were long-term dental avoiders (six years and 13 years) but, following treatment, both obtained dental care at regular intervals.

Summary and Recommendations The methods we have discussed have all been found helpful in reducing dental fear. Of these methods, a combined approach (modeling and relaxation) has produced the most impressive results with very fearful, avoidant patients.

Which of these methods should you use with your fearful patients? Choice of method depends on several factors, including space, availability of equipment and personnel, and the fearfulness of the individual patient in question.

---

* *These figures are based on the application of these treatment methods with patients who, for the most part, suffered long-term fear so intense that it prevented them from even appearing in a dental office. Thus, we would expect higher rates of improvement using these methods with patients who are at least able to present themselves in the dental office.*

With highly fearful patients (those who obtain a score of four to five on the Dental Fear Survey, or a score of 15 or greater on the Corah Dental Anxiety Scale), we suggest that the following sequence of activities be made available to the patient if video equipment, space for the equipment, operatory space, and personnel are available.

Visit #1 Provide a cassette audiotape with relaxation instructions and a desensitization hierarchy for at-home use. Instruct the patient to listen to the entire tape daily until the next visit. Schedule the next visit within seven to ten days.

Visit #2 Have the patient listen to audiotaped relaxation instructions, then view a modeling film. Allow the patient to sit in the reception area for 15 to 20 minutes, then in the operatory for 15 to 20 minutes. If a dental assistant cannot remain with the patient in the operatory, she should check with him frequently. Prophylaxis can be done at this visit if the patient agrees, or he may defer this to the next visit.

Visit #3 Allow the patient to listen to audiotaped relaxation instructions through earphones during prophylaxis and/or treatment. At subsequent visits, the patient can be offered the choice of listening to the relaxation tape or playing a video game (see Chapter Five).

If video equipment is not available, employ the same sequence of events described above, omitting the modeling procedure. In either case, outline the entire sequence to the patient before beginning. However, be sure to make it clear that, while the entire sequence is available to him, he can omit steps if he feels he is ready to proceed at a faster pace.

For example, at the second visit the patient may report significant improvement and elect to omit one or more of the steps scheduled for this visit. The patient is, of course, the best judge of his own level of fear and you can safely follow his lead.

Patients who are less fearful can simply be given the at-home tape and can then listen to taped relaxation instructions at subsequent visits. If additional procedures should prove necessary, they can be employed as needed.

We believe that all patients, regardless of level of fear, should be offered an opportunity to listen to a relaxation tape (or play video games, if available) while in the chair. Even the low-fear patient becomes bored and restless during lengthy treatment appointments and the tapes or games can help relieve boredom and restlessness.

Below are some questions dentists commonly ask about treatment of the fearful patient.

Q: Are these formal treatment methods really necessary? Isn't it sufficient if the dentist is compassionate, understanding, and proceeds slowly and cautiously?

A: The dentist's ability to communicate concern and understanding is, of course, an important ingredient. With some mildly fearful patients, this may be sufficient to reduce anxiety. However, more fearful patients often require additional assistance. One recent study[24] showed that, while seeing a dentist who was chosen to provide a nonaversive experience was helpful to some patients, it was significantly less effective than the formal treatment methods used with other groups of patients.

Q: Should the dentist limit himself to treating mildly fearful patients or can he appropriately offer fear-reduction treatment to any fearful patient, regardless of level of fear?

A: It is safe to say that if a patient arrives in your office, he is not overwhelmed by his fear. Therefore, it seems ethically defensible to offer fear-reduction treatment programs to any and all of your fearful patients.

Q: Under what circumstances should a patient be referred to a psychologist for treatment of dental fear?

A: It is appropriate to refer a patient for such treatment if your treatment program fails to reduce his fear enough to enable him to undergo dental treatment without excessive discomfort and anxiety.

REFERENCES

1. Crockett, B. "Dental survey: Southeastern State College." *Okla S Dent A J* 55:25, 1965.
2. Freedson, E. and Feldman, J. J. "The public looks at dental care." *Am Dent A J* 57:325, 1958.
3. Kleinknecht, R. A.; Klepac, R. K.; Alexander, D. A. "Origins and characteristics of fear of dentistry." *Am Dent A J* 86:842, 1973.
4. Ingersoll, B. D.; Ingersoll, T. G.; McCutcheon, W. R.; Seime, R. J. "Behavioral aspects of dental practice: A national survey." Unpublished manuscript, West Virginia University School of Dentistry, 1979.
5. Kleinknecht, R. A. "Dental fear assessment." In *Behavioral Dentistry: Proceedings of the First National Conference.* edited by B. Ingersoll, R. Seime, W. McCutcheon. Morgantown, W. Va.: West Virginia University, 1977.
6. Lautch, H. "Dental phobia." *Brit J Psych* 119:151, 1971.
7. Shoben, E. J. Jr, and Borland, L. "An empirical study of the etiology of dental fears." *J Clin Psychol* 10:171, 1954.
8. Kleinknecht, R. A. "Fear of dentistry: Its development, measurement and implications." In *Advances in Behavioral Research in Dentistry,* edited by P. Weinstein. Seattle: University of Washington, 1978.

9. Morgan, P.; Wright, L.; Ingersoll, B. S.; Seime R. J. "Children's perception of the dental experience." *J Dent Child* 47:243, 1980.

10. Corah, N. L. "Development of a dental anxiety scale." *J Dent Res* 48:596, 1969.

11. Corah, N. L.; Gale, E. N.; Illig, S. J. "Assessment of a dental anxiety scale." *Am Dent A J* 97:816, 1978.

12. Corah, N. L.; Bissell, G. D.; Illig, S. J. "Effect of perceived control on stress reduction in adult dental patients." *J Dent Res* 57:74, 1978.

13. Stricker, G. and Howitt, J. W. "Physiological recording during simulated dental appointments." *NYS Dent J* 31:204, 1965.

14. Kleinknecht, R. A. and Bernstein, D. A. "The assessment of dental fear." *Behav Therapy* 9:626, 1978.

15. Kleinknecht, R. A. and Bernstein, D. A. "Fear assessment in the dental office." In *Clinical Research in Behavioral Dentistry: Proceedings of the Second National Conference on Behavioral Dentistry*, edited by B. D. Ingersoll and W. R. McCutcheon. Morgantown, W. Va.: West Virginia University, 1979.

16. Jackson, E. "Managing dental fears: A tentative code of practice." *J Oral Med* 29:96, 1974.

17. Wright, G. Z. *Behavior Management in Dentistry for Children*. Philadelphia: W. B. Saunders, 1975.

18. Hirschman, R. "Physiological feedback and stress reduction." In B. Ingersoll (chair): *Behavioral Approaches to Dental Fear, Pain, and Stress*. Symposium presented at the meeting of the Society of Behavioral Medicine, New York, 1980.

19. Hirschman, R.; Young, D.; Nelson, C. "Physiologically based techniques for stress reduction." In *Clinical Research in Behavioral Dentistry: Proceedings of the Second National Conference on Behavioral Dentistry*, edited by B. D. Ingersoll and W. R. McCutcheon. Morgantown, W. Va.: West Virginia University, 1979.

20. Wolpe, J. *Psychotherapy by Reciprocal Inhibition*. Stanford: Stanford University Press, 1958.

21. Gale, E. N. and Ayer, W. A. "Treatment of dental phobias." *Am Dent A J* 78:1304, 1969.

22. Klepac, R. K. "Successful treatment of avoidance of dentistry by desensitization or by increasing pain tolerance." *J Behav Therapy and Experimental Psych* 6:307, 1975.

23. Shaw, D. W. and Thoreson, C. E. "Effects of modeling and desensitization in reducing dental phobia." *J Counsel Psychol* 20:415, 1974.

24. Bernstein, D. A. and Kleinknecht, R. A. "Comparative evaluation of three social-learning approaches to the reduction of dental fear." In *Clinical Research in Behavioral Dentistry: Proceedings of the Second National Conference on Behavioral Dentistry*, edited by B. D. Ingersoll and W. R. McCutcheon. Morgantown, W. Va.: West Virginia University, 1979.

25. Illig, S. J.; Corah, N. L.; Gale, E. N. "Anxiety correlates of dental stress reduction." Paper presented at the 56th International Association for Dental Research, Washington, DC, March 16, 1978.

26. Machen, J. and Johnson, R. "Desensitization, model learning, and the dental behavior of children." *J Dent Res* 53:83, 1974.

27. Melamed, B. G. "Preparing children for dental treatment: Effects of film modeling." In *Clinical Research in Behavioral Dentistry: Proceedings of the Second National*

Conference on Behavioral Dentistry, edited by B. D. Ingersoll and W. R. McCutcheon. Morgantown, W. Va.: West Virginia University, 1979.

28. Wroblewski, P. F.; Jacob, T.; Rehm, L. P. "The contribution of relaxation to symbolic modeling in the modification of dental fears." *Behav Res and Therapy* 15:113, 1977.

29. Kleinknecht, R. A. and Bernstein, D. A. "Short-term treatment of dental avoidance." *J Behav Therapy and Experimental Psych* 10:311, 1979.

5

The Management of Pain and Discomfort

The practicing dentist encounters pain on a daily basis. For him, it is an unavoidable fact of professional life—an "inherent handicap," as we noted in an earlier chapter. Sometimes, of course, pain presents in a beneficial form, as when it prompts a patient to seek needed care. More commonly, pain is an unfortunate by-product of dentistry, hindering treatment and causing patients to fear and avoid dental care.

The diagnosis of acute pain and discomfort can be a source of great professional satisfaction to the dentist. However, the dentist is less likely to achieve success with chronic pain problems, as they present fewer opportunities for technical remediation. In such cases, especially when no organic cause for the pain can be identified, the dentist can easily become bewildered and frustrated.

Although exciting discoveries have been made in pain research in recent years, there is much about pain that remains a puzzle to the researcher and clinician alike. Pain is as old as man, yet researchers have not been able to arrive at a satisfactory definition of pain. Each of us knows what it is to suffer pain, but it is not a simple matter to define or quantify pain because it is a complex, subjective phenomenon.

Our understanding of pain has been both helped and hindered by a tendency to focus on its neurophysiological aspects. This approach has advanced our scientific knowledge, but, at the same time, it has drawn attention away from the psychological aspects of the pain experience. In the search for new surgical and pharmacological methods to relieve pain, psychological methods have, until recently, been sadly overlooked.

Thus, although the clinical value of suggestion and placebo has been apparent for many years, we have failed to capitalize on these effects in a systematic, intentional fashion. Hypnosis, too, has suffered a similar fate. Reports of the successful use of hypnosis to induce anesthesia for surgery date back to the early nineteenth century, yet hypnotists have usually been viewed as charlatans. Only in recent years has hypnosis been considered a subject worthy of serious scientific study.

Neglect of psychological approaches to the treatment of pain is particularly unfortunate from a clinical perspective, as these methods are sometimes successful when other methods have failed, especially in cases of chronic pain. In addition, the effectiveness of pharmacological approaches can be enhanced by appropriate psychological interventions.

As we will explain, psychological factors are intrinsic to the pain experience. Pain cannot be experienced—indeed, pain cannot even be said to exist—independent of these factors. It is obvious, then, that expert knowledge of the physiological aspects of pain is not sufficient to understand pain or to treat patients in pain. The admonition to "treat the total person, not just the pain" makes little sense to the clinician who conceptualizes pain only in physiological terms. Unfortunately, dental education, with its emphasis on basic sciences and technical skill acquisition, often produces clinicians who are not well acquainted with the importance of psychological factors in pain. Rather, the dental student's training naturally produces clinicians who are oriented principally toward a physiological, or disease model, approach to conceptualizing and treating pain. We will discuss the advantages and disadvantages of this model in the following section.

CONCEPTUALIZING AND DEFINING PAIN

The Disease Model: Pain Reflects Organic Pathology

According to the disease model of pain, the origin of pain lies in tissue damage or organic pathology. If the causative agent can be identified and removed or treated by surgical, pharmacological, or mechanical means, the pain will cease.

In clinical work, this approach has often produced beneficial results. Many patients with acute pain have obtained effective and efficient relief through surgical or pharmacological means.

However, a strict adherence to the disease model of pain, to the exclusion of other approaches, is shortsighted and carries serious risks. It can lead, for example, to an overreliance on surgical or pharmacological methods when other approaches might be more effective or entail less risk—or both. Certainly, the evidence indicates that this is the case with chronic pain. Although some patients have benefited from surgical treatment for pain, surgical methods for the relief of chronic pain have proved generally disappointing. Surgical procedures often must be very extensive to produce relief, but the more extensive the surgery, the greater the likelihood that other functions will be lost. In addition, it is not uncommon for pain to return after surgery. As one authority has noted:

> Almost every possible type of nervous connection from the periphery to the sensory cortex has been surgically cut without successfully permanently abolishing the pain. No matter what technique is used, the percentage of failures is significant.[1]

We must remember, too, that surgery is never without an element of risk. This is also the case when drugs are used to treat pain, especially chronic pain. With drugs, the clinician must contend with the problems of increased tolerance, addiction, side effects, and toxicity.

There are additional dangers if we rely solely on a disease model of pain. The clinician, confronted with a pain for which no organic cause can be found, may conclude that the patient is malingering or that the pain is "all in the patient's head." Blaming the patient for his pain may relieve the dentist's frustration, but it does nothing to relieve the patient's pain.

Finally, the disease model of pain simply cannot account for much of what we know about pain. The model implies, for example, that the intensity of pain experienced is directly proportional to the amount of tissue damage sustained or noxious stimulation applied. This is not always the case. We know that soldiers wounded in battle may report little or no pain despite extensive tissue damage. Similarly, an athlete may be seriously injured during a heated contest but may not even notice the pain until the game has ended. Conversely, pain may occur in the absence of detectable tissue damage, or it may persist long after injured tissue has healed.

The examples given above indicate that pain cannot be defined solely in physiological terms, nor can it be reduced to the level of a simple sensory experience or sensation. Indeed, as one pioneer in the study of pain points out:

> It is surely true that there is no such thing as a pure sensation, all sensations having been modified probably at the subcortical level before they erupt into consciousness and certainly modified after erupting into consciousness by conditioning, significance, meaning.[2]

Pain, then, like any sensory event, must be processed by the individual who experiences it. Melzack, co-author of the well-known "gate control theory" discussed below, has stated:

> Pain (is) a perceptual experience whose quality and intensity is influenced by the past history of the individual, the meaning he gives

to the pain-producing situation, and by his "state of mind" at the moment . . . (thus) pain becomes a function of the whole individual, including his present thoughts and fears, as well as his hopes for the future.[3]

We see that the perception of pain depends not only on the physical stimulus but on a host of other variables, including the individual's past experiences and his current physical and emotional state. The psychological aspect of pain, then, is inseparable from the experience of pain.

Gate Control Theory: An Alternative Model

How can these different aspects of pain be linked together? How do the psychological factors relate to the physiological events of pain? We think that gate control theory, developed by Melzack and Wall,[4] provides a framework within which these questions can best be answered and the psychological aspect of pain can best be understood. The dentist, trained in the biological sciences, may also come to a greater appreciation of the psychological factors in pain if he is aware of the body of neurophysiological evidence for the role of these factors.

Although the exact physiological mechanisms underlying the theory have not yet all been established and the theory itself is considered controversial, gate control theory has proved extremely useful in its ability to organize information about pain and to explain many of the puzzling aspects of pain perception. Perhaps more importantly, gate control theory has exciting implications for the treatment and control of pain.

Gate control theory is briefly summarized in the following sections. The reader interested in further information is referred to Ronald Melzack's fascinating book, *The Puzzle of Pain.* *

Neurophysiological Processes Sensory nerve fibers, which conduct nerve impulses from peripheral receptor sites to the spinal cord, include large-diameter, myelinated fibers which transmit the nerve impulse very rapidly, and smaller fibers along which the nerve impulse is transmitted more slowly. Large-diameter fibers are involved with the transmission of non-painful tactile stimulation, while small fibers are associated with receptors which respond to high-intensity stimulation (such as crushing or burning).

Nerve impulses transmitted along sensory nerve fibers enter the spinal cord at the *dorsal horns* and activate dorsal horn transmission cells (*T cells*). These T cells project information to wide areas of the brain via several spinal cord pathways. *When the total output of the T cells reaches or exceeds a critical level, pain is experienced.*

---

* *New York: Basic Books, 1973.*

What factors determine the total output of the T cells? We know that activation of the T cells depends in part on the total number of active sensory nerve fibers and their rate of firing.

In addition, Melzack and Wall hypothesize that a *gate control mechanism* in the substantia gelatinosa of dorsal horns regulates the amount of activity in the T cells. This gate control mechanism is influenced both by afferent nerve impulses from peripheral sensory nerves and by efferent nerve impulses descending from the brain.

Afferent Influences on the Gate   Afferent influence on the gate depends on the relative amount of activity in large, rapidly conducting fibers and in small, slower fibers. Volleys of nerve impulses transmitted along large fibers *inhibit* the activity of the T cells, *reducing* the amount of information they transmit and "closing the gate." Nerve impulses transmitted along small fibers, on the other hand, have an *excitatory* effect on the T cells; activity is *increased,* "opening the gate."

This explains why mild sensory stimulation, such as rubbing, scratching, or vibration, applied to an area adjacent to an injury might bring some relief from pain. Mild stimulation activates a greater number of large fibers, producing inhibition of T cells and a closing, or partial closing, of the gate. Conversely, damage to large peripheral nerve fibers through injury or disease alters the ratio of large to small fibers in favor of small fibers. The net effect is excitation of the T cells and an opening of the gate.

Efferent Influences on the Gate   The gate control mechanism is also influenced by activity in nerve fibers descending from the brain. Melzack and Wall hypothesize that incoming signals from the periphery, transmitted through rapidly conducting spinal cord systems, act to trigger selective central processes of *attention, emotion,* and *memory.* This, in turn, activates a number of efferent systems which act directly on the gate to modify activity in the T cells.

In short, central mechanisms serve to evaluate, then diminish or enhance, incoming signals arriving at the dorsal horn. These central mechanisms are activated so rapidly that they can evaluate and modify incoming signals before the individual actually experiences pain. As Melzack points out:

> These rapidly conducting ascending and descending systems can thus account for the fact that psychological processes play a powerful role in determining the quality and intensity of pain.[4]

What factors determine whether the action of the central trigger mechanism will diminish or, alternately, enhance the incoming signals? The central control mechanisms are influenced by factors such as the current emotional state of the organism, ongoing activity and competing stimuli, and previous experience. Anxiety, for example, can serve to open the gate, while excitement or distraction may cause a closing, or partial closing, of the gate.

The extent to which central mechanisms are able to effect the gate depends, too, on the temporal and spatial qualities of input patterns from the periphery. Certain kinds of pain which rise slowly in intensity may allow time for cognitive activities to act on the gate, while other types of pain, such as cardiac pain, rise too quickly in intensity to allow this.

Summary   In summary, the total integrated output of the T cells is regulated by:

1. The total number of active peripheral nerve fibers and their rate of firing
2. The ratio of large-diameter to small-diameter fibers firing
3. Activity of the central structures

When the total output of the T cells exceeds a critical level, the action system for pain is triggered and the individual perceives and responds to pain. Melzack concludes that:

> These ascending and descending interactions present a picture of dynamic, modifiable processes in which inputs impinge on a continually active nervous system that is already the repository of the individual's past history, expectations, and value systems. This . . . means that the input patterns evoked by injury can be modulated by other sensory inputs or by descending influences, which may thereby determine the quality and intensity of the eventual experience.[4]

Gate control theory, as we have noted, has proved especially useful in directing attention toward new methods of control, particularly psychological methods. In addition, gate control theory "fits" much of what we know about pain. Finally, this model avoids a narrow focus on physiological events and reminds us that, as clinicians, we do not treat *pain* — we treat *patients who experience pain*.

Defining Pain

We are now ready to present a working definition of pain. We have adopted Mersky and Spear's well-known operational definition of pain as: ". . . an unpleasant experience which we primarily associate with tissue damage or describe in terms of such damage, or both."[5] This definition offers a number of advantages:

- It emphasizes the association of pain with tissue damage, but it avoids the incorrect assumption of a direct, fixed relationship between the two.
- It does not limit us to a search for organic causes of pain; instead, it allows us to view pain as the result of numerous etiological factors.
- It leads away from a narrow focus on surgical and pharmacological treatment methods toward a broader consideration of other means of managing pain.
- It avoids the artificial and dangerous dichotomy between "real" pain and "psychological" pain. It forces us to recognize that a pain is a pain, whether its origins lie in a wound, a stressful day at the office, or an unconscious desire to avoid an unpleasant task.

In summary, this definition recognizes the neurophysiological/organic aspects of pain ("tissue damage"), but it also reminds us that pain is a personal and subjective event ("unpleasant experience") involving thoughts and emotions ("associates").

PSYCHOLOGICAL FACTORS IN PAIN PERCEPTION AND BEHAVIOR

We have stressed the central role of psychological factors in the perception of pain and in the individual's behavior in response to pain. We now turn to an examination of these factors and the ways in which they influence the pain experience. In this section, factors related to acute pain are emphasized; chronic pain is discussed in greater detail in a later section.

Learning: The Role of Experience
The idea that one must "learn" to feel and express pain may seem odd, but we know that gross interference with normal developmental processes may interfere with the ability to respond appropriately to painful events. Dogs reared in complete isolation, for example, fail to respond normally to such painful stimuli as pinpricks and burning matches. These animals show no apparent distress, nor do they learn to avoid the flame or pin, even after many trials.[6]

Ethnic and Cultural Background Cultural differences in reaction to pain also reflect the role of learning in pain behavior. Although the level of stimulation at which *sensation* is first detected is uniform for all people, individuals vary considerably in the amount of stimulation required before they (a) report feeling pain; (b) show overt signs of pain, such as grimacing or withdrawing from the stimulation; and, (c) refuse to tolerate additional stimulation (in the laboratory setting).

Many studies have reported differences among ethnic and cultural groups in their responses to pain. People of Mediterranean origin, such as Italians and Jews, for example, are apt to *report* pain before people of northern European descent and to *tolerate* less intense levels of laboratory-induced pain before refusing to continue.[7,8]

These differences in pain-related behavior reflect differences in ethnic attitudes towards pain. Some ethnic groups encourage stoic attitudes and behavior. Among other groups, a person in pain is expected to express pain responses openly and receives sympathy and attention for this behavior.

As cultural patterns are transmitted in large part by the family, we might expect the family to be an important source of early learning about pain perception and appropriate behavior in response to pain. Family members not only serve as examples, or models, of how pain should be expressed; by their responses to the person in pain, they actively support or discourage particular patterns of pain behavior. Sometimes this teaching is quite obvious, as when a child is told, "Big boys don't cry." At other times it is more subtle (but no less powerful), as when an ill or injured child receives extra attention and affection.

The role of the family assumes special importance with chronic pain patients. Families of such patients unwittingly but almost inevitably contribute to the maintenance of chronic pain conditions by their well-meaning attempts to provide sympathy and support. In the treatment of chronic pain, the role of the family is considered so critical that at least one well-known authority on the treatment of chronic pain refuses to accept patients for treatment unless their family also agrees to participate in the treatment plan.[9]

Age and Sex Differences   According to folklore, women are fragile and sensitive; men are "tougher" than women and can "take more pain." Health care professionals—who are, after all, members of their culture and, therefore, influenced by cultural norms—seem to have accepted these stereotypes. For example, research has shown that among postoperative patients, women are likely to be given pain drugs earlier than men.[10] In addition, men must complain more than women about pain before being given pain medication.[11]

At first glance, laboratory studies would seem to support this notion. Most studies of *pain tolerance* (the amount of painful stimulation a person is willing to tolerate before refusing to continue) have found that men are willing to tolerate more pain than women. However, an equal number of studies have demonstrated that when *pain threshold* (the point at which the person reports feeling pain) is used as a measure, men and women do not differ. This suggests that sex differences in pain behavior probably reflect the influence of learning rather than differences in physiology. In our culture, as in many others, behavior that is acceptable in a woman is not considered appropriate in a man. Little girls learn that crying about a skinned knee often brings sympathy and comfort from others; little boys are told to "act like a man" and that "only babies cry."

Learning may also be related to differences in pain behavior between younger and older persons. Again, studies suggest that pain threshold does not change with age but that older people may be more reluctant to label a sensation as painful.

Implications for the Dentist   The studies we have discussed reflect group data. While such studies allow us to make probability statements, the accuracy of predictions concerning a specific individual is limited. That is, we can say, "It is likely that our older, male patients will tolerate higher levels of painful stimulation without complaint than will our younger, female patients, but we cannot say exactly how young Mrs. Smith or old Mr. Jones will react to pain."

The data from these studies should remind us, however, that we are largely dependent on verbal and motor behavior when we attempt to assess pain and that these measures are not always reliable indicators. Just as the absence of demonstrable organic pathology should not lead us to conclude that the patient should not feel pain, so should we also be cautious in assuming that the absence of complaints and grimaces indicates an absence of pain. The cardinal rule here is: If you have any reason to suspect that your patient is uncomfortable or in pain, *ask!*

Situational Factors in Pain Perception

A person's past experiences are certainly important in determining his responses to pain in any given situation. However, various aspects of the situation itself also contribute to pain perception.

Attention   A person who is caught up in an intensely absorbing or exciting experience may not even notice painful stimulation when it occurs. It may not be until later, when the excitement and high emotion have passed, that he feels pain and realizes that he has suffered a serious injury.

People suffering from acutely or chronically painful conditions very often report that the pain is much worse at night. During the day a variety of events and activities distract them, but in the quiet hours of the night there are no distractions, and their attention is focused on their pain.

These examples illustrate the important role of attention in pain perception. In general, when a person's attention is directed toward painful stimulation, that stimulation is experienced as more intense. Measures which serve to distract or redirect attention contribute to pain reduction. Among laboratory subjects, the use of the word "pain" in the instructions leads them to rate stimulation as more painful than when the word is not used.[12] Conversely, when subjects are instructed to focus their attention on such distracting material as slides, stories, movies, and word and number tasks, pain perception is reduced.[13,14]

In the dental operatory, distraction in the form of white noise and music has been found to be an effective pain-reducing tactic for many patients.[15] This approach, known as "audio analgesia," did not live up to early claims of complete pain suppression for all patients. However, when accompanied by strong suggestion concerning its beneficial effects from a dentist who could relate well to his patients, audio analgesia proved sufficiently distracting to provide a measure of pain relief for many patients.[4]

More recently, the use of television programs and video games have been used as distractors in the dental operatory. Such methods are promising adjuncts to current means of relieving discomfort and pain during dental treatment

Anxiety   Anxiety is a basic ingredient of acute pain. The relationship is simple and clear-cut: Increased anxiety results in greater sensitivity to pain and, conversely, methods which reduce anxiety also reduce pain.

In the laboratory, low-anxious subjects rate sensations produced by radiant heat and electric shock as less painful than do subjects in whom anxiety is experimentally induced.[12] Similarly, people who fear dental treatment rate the pain experienced during experimental tooth shock as far more intense than do people who describe themselves as low in dental fear.[16] These studies are of particular importance to the dentist, because they indicate that the anxious patient who winces at the anesthetic injection and groans at every touch is not just a "big baby." Such patients actually experience the procedures as more painful than other patients who are less fearful of dental treatment.

Numerous lines of evidence also indicate that when anxiety is reduced, the intensity of pain experienced is also reduced. In the clinical setting, when preoperative anxiety is reduced through instructions, explanation, and support, patients require far less postoperative pain medication and are ready for discharge earlier than patients who are not given such preparation.[17]

The effectiveness of pain-relieving medication is also directly related to the sufferer's anxiety level. Morphine reduces pain if anxiety level is high but has little or no effect if the patient is not anxious.[12] Similarly, the effectiveness of placebos in reducing pain appears directly related to the level of anxiety associated with the pain.[18]

What factors contribute to increased anxiety and, hence, to increased pain perception? In the clinical setting, the most important variables are:

- the extent to which the patient understands and can predict what is going to happen to him

- the amount of control the patient believes he has over the situation
- the meaning the patient attaches to the pain situation.

As we noted in Chapter 4, *unpredictability* of a painful event heightens anxiety and pain perception. Patients who do not know what to expect usually anticipate the worst. When this anticipatory anxiety is reduced by providing clear explanations and information, laboratory subjects and clinical patients alike report reductions in pain. Accurate descriptions of procedures to be performed and the sensations that will accompany them help the patient to prepare for uncomfortable or painful events and to cope more effectively with them. An important component in modeling procedures, discussed in Chapter 4, is that they serve to make clear to the patient exactly what to expect. The Tell-Show-Do method, widely endorsed by pedodontists, attempts to achieve this through verbal means but is somewhat less effective than modeling procedures. Films, of course, are an excellent means of conveying a great amount of detailed information with a minimum of time and effort on the dentist's part. A variety of such films are available commercially.

Prediction is closely related to control. A particularly frightening aspect of clinical pain is the sufferer's feeling that he cannot control the pain. Laboratory subjects who control the onset and termination of painful stimulation, rate the pain as less intense than is the case when the experimenter retains control.[12] Therefore, it is important that patients be given as much control over potentially painful situations as is possible. In addition to the commonly used instruction, "Raise your hand if you would like me to stop," patients can also be given control over length and frequency of appointments, type of anesthetic, and alternate treatment plans.

In many cases, actual control over the situation is not exercised—the perception of control is sufficient to calm the patient. This probably accounts for the fact that few patients ever actually act on the dentist's suggestion concerning the hand signal. Of course, as Jackson notes, if the patient should signal you, stop immediately.

The meaning of the situation also affects anxiety in important ways. During World War II, H. K. Beecher, the Harvard anesthesiologist well-known for his extensive studies of the relationship between pain and anxiety, observed many soldiers who were wounded during the intense shelling of the beach at Anzio. He noted that, of 215 men who were seriously wounded, only 25 percent requested pain medication. In contrast, in Beecher's civilian practice, over 80 percent of surgical patients with comparable wounds made under anesthesia requested medication to relieve the pain.[19] The significance of the wound, rather than the extent of tissue damage, appeared responsible for the difference. For the soldiers, a serious wound meant a ticket to safety, but for the civilians, surgery was a frightening, disruptive event in their lives.

How does the meaning of the situation affect the patient undergoing dental treatment? The meaning attached to the situation depends, of course, on the individual patient, but it seems safe to say that for some patients (even those who are low in dental fear), the need for dental treatment represents failure or defeat; they have failed in the care of their teeth. Some patients feel a sense of helplessness and even anger, as if they were "at the mercy" of their untrustworthy teeth. When a patient replies to the question, "What brings you here today?" with, "a toothache" or "a broken filling," he may also be expressing the uncomfortable feeling that he had no choice —he was forced to seek care.

You can help such patients view dental treatment in a more positive light by getting them to perceive their own role as active and constructive instead of passive and helpless. Begin by praising the patient's decision to come in for treatment, even if it is obvious that he postponed the decision well past the point of good sense. When you say, "I'm really glad you came in today," you imply, "You made an intelligent decision." On the other hand, if you say, "If you hadn't waited so long, this wouldn't have happened," you are clearly telling the patient, "You behaved stupidly." No one enjoys receiving criticism. With a patient who is already somewhat resentful, such tactics can only add fuel to his negative feelings.

Throughout the session, gently stress the positive. If the patient asks, "Can you save my tooth?" a blunt, "I don't know" in response is unsettling and can increase his anxiety. It is more reassuring (and equally honest) to say, "I will certainly do everything I can." Emphasize the benefits the patient will experience as a result of his decision to seek care. The patient will probably feel better; he may even look better—remember to remind him of these benefits.

In summary, factors such as understanding and control over the situation and the meaning of the situation influence anxiety and, hence, the subjective experience of pain. Measures which serve to give the patient a clear understanding of what will happen to him and which provide him with a feeling of some control help to reduce anxiety. Anxiety is also reduced when the patient is able to perceive some positive aspects of the situation. Additional methods for reducing anxiety and pain perception are discussed in the following section.

REDUCTION OF ACUTE PAIN AND DISCOMFORT

The practicing dentist today has a large armamentarium of excellent pharmacologic methods to reduce pain. Psychological methods are not intended as replacements for these methods. Rather, they should be viewed as adjuncts—useful tools which can enhance the effectiveness of pain-relieving drugs and can help make dental treatment a more positive experience, not only for the patient, but for the dentist and his staff as well.

Many of the methods discussed in this section are already in widespread use among practicing dentists. In fact, the dental profession has for many years led other health care professions in their search for, and utilization of, nonpharmacologic methods to reduce pain and fear and promote patient comfort. Dentists, as we shall discuss, have pioneered the use of clinical hypnosis and it is largely due to their efforts that hypnosis has gained current widespread acceptance among the health care professions.

As in other areas of behavioral dentistry, definitive research concerning the effectiveness of these methods in the clinical setting is not yet abundant. The bulk of the evidence available to date, however, strongly suggests that these methods are of considerable merit with many patients. By presenting a detailed discussion of these methods, we hope to clarify some misconceptions and to encourage the use of these methods on a broader and more systematic basis in clinical dentistry.

Relaxation

The central role of anxiety in pain perception suggests that relaxation procedures might be of use in controlling pain. Among laboratory subjects, relaxation training has been shown to be an effective means of increasing tolerance for radiant-heat and pressure-algometer stimulation.[20] Clinically, relaxation has been taught to patients with myofascial pain dysfunction syndrome (MPD), among whom excessive tension in masticatory muscles is a major factor in pain and dysfunction. Of 11 patients, only five who were also depressed did not benefit; the remainder obtained good results.[21]

As we noted in our discussion of fearful patients, relaxation alone is not sufficient to produce good results with all patients. However, when combined with other methods, it is a useful adjunctive strategy.

Suggestion and Placebo

The use of suggestion to relieve pain and promote healing is by no means new. At the dawn of civilization, high priests used elaborate ceremonies, rituals, and incantations to heighten the patient's expectation for recovery. These methods were sometimes surprisingly effective, as evidenced by the awe in which priests and shamans were held and by their power and status in society.

In our discussion of "audio analgesia" in an earlier section, we noted that this technique was found effective in reducing pain and discomfort when accompanied by strong suggestion to that effect. Further evidence of the powerful influence of suggestion on pain perception comes from studies on the effectiveness of *placebos*.

The word "placebo" is Latin for "I shall please." The term "placebo effect" refers to the effects of any substance or procedure which is known to have no specific therapeutic effects on the condition for which it is being administered.

Placebo effects can sometimes be quite dramatic. In a classic example of this, ipecac, a known emetic, brought relief to people suffering from nausea and vomiting.[22] More closely related to the dental field is a study in which placebo appliances, used with patients suffering myofascial pain dysfunction, resulted in remission or noticeable improvement in symptoms in more than 40 percent of the group.[23]

Among patients suffering postoperative pain, about 75 percent obtain significant relief from morphine, but about 35 percent obtain a comparable degree of relief from placebos, suggesting that about half of the effect of morphine may be a placebo effect.[24] This reminds us of an important but often overlooked point; even drugs which are pharmacologically active have a placebo component. Accompanying the administration of any drug or procedure is the suggestion, implicit or explicit, that it will produce beneficial effects. The stronger and more enthusiastic the suggestion and the greater the patient's trust in and respect for the professional who prescribes the treatment, the greater the placebo effect. The patient's belief that something is being done for him, and his expectation of relief, may reduce his anxiety and, hence, his pain.

Indeed, placebo effectiveness is greatest when pain is very severe and when the patient is highly anxious.[25] Among laboratory subjects, placebos are ten times less effective than is the case with individuals whose pain is of pathologic origin.[25] This striking difference can be attributed to the differences between the two groups in anxiety. The laboratory subject knows that his pain will be limited in duration and intensity and that he will not suffer permanent injury, disfigurement, or death; the clinical patient has no such assurance.

The studies cited above illustrate an important point about placebo response. The tendency to respond to a placebo does not appear to be related to any inherent characteristics of the individual, such as personality attributes. Rather, placebo reactivity seems to be situationally determined and the individual's response is determined by the interaction of several factors. Factors which have been found important in the dental setting, specifically, include the enthusiasm with which the dentist or dental technician endorsed the placebo and the warmth displayed by the dentist or technician toward the patient.[26]

The placebo effect is usually considered a nuisance by researchers attempting to evaluate new drugs and procedures. It is also viewed with suspicion among clinicians, many of whom erroneously believe that if a patient is helped by a placebo, his pain was not "real" in the first place. Of course, this belief not only reflects an incomplete understanding of the nature of pain; it flies in the face of evidence that placebos can produce measurable physiological effects such as changes in corticosteroid levels.[26]

Nevertheless, these factors probably account, in large part, for the fact that little has been done in the way of systematic and intentional utilization of the placebo effect to benefit the patient in pain. Of course, the use of deliberate deception is not ethically defensible (except, perhaps, in certain unique cases). However, since the placebo effect is present in all treatment procedures, and since this effect can be influenced positively or negatively by the personality and behavior of the health care professional, the wise dentist will strive to maximize positive effects with all of his patients.

Hypnosis

Hypnosis, in its more modern form, can be traced to the late 18th century, when Franz Anton Mesmer, a Viennese physician, intrigued Parisians with displays of "magnetism." Although Mesmer and his theory of magnetism were discredited by a royal commission appointed to study mesmerism, there is no doubt that Mesmer did achieve some dramatic, and often therapeutic, effects.

Reports of painless surgery performed with mesmerism, or hypnosis, as it later came to be called, date back to the early 19th century. In 1829, for example, a French surgeon named Cloquet used hypnosis in the reportedly painless removal of a patient's cancerous breast.

Hypnosis was also used in dentistry during this period. The first documented use of hypnosis in dentistry was that of Oudet, who, in 1820, reported extracting teeth using hypnosis as the only anesthetic.

Despite many other reports of the effectiveness of hypnosis in reducing or eliminating pain associated with surgery, the report of the French royal commission led most people to view hypnosis with extreme skepticism. Hypnosis did not achieve scientific respectability and, with the development of chemical anesthesia in the early 20th century, interest in hypnosis all but vanished.

In recent years, there has been a revival of interest in hypnosis within the medical and dental professions. The number of books and articles devoted to the topic has increased markedly and two national societies concerned exclusively with hypnosis have been formed.* Each society publishes a journal and sponsors workshops and educational programs on hypnosis.

Interestingly, dentists have played a major role in the modern revival of interest in hypnosis. Perhaps because of the types of problems they must

---

* *The American Society for Clinical Hypnosis, 2400 East Devon Avenue—Suite 218, Des Plaines, Illinois 60018; The Society for Clinical and Experimental Hypnosis, 129-A Kings Park Drive, Liverpool, New York 13088.*

handle on a daily basis, dentists have pioneered the clinical use of hypnosis and have found it to be a valuable tool with a broad range of applications. As listed in the workshop syllabus of the Education and Research Foundation of the American Society of Clinical Hypnosis,[27] these applications include the following:

- For the nervous, jittery, apprehensive patient
- For those who set up defense mechanisms to postpone actual work
- For the functional or psychosomatic gagger
- For thumbsucking
- For bruxism
- For better control of hemorrhage and salivation
- To reinforce instructions for oral hygiene
- For those who refuse anesthesia because of hypodermic needles
- As a substitute for chemical anesthesia, in certain cases
- for psychological problems arising from dentures and orthodontic appliances

Despite this impressive list, and despite the fact that courses in hypnosis are available in many dental schools and continuing education programs, the use of hypnosis among dentists is not as widespread as might be expected. This may be due in part to the mistaken belief that the use of hypnosis increases the time needed for the dental visit. In fact, the opposite is true: work can proceed more easily and quickly with a relaxed and cooperative patient than with one who is tense and apprehensive. A practitioner who is skilled in the use of hypnosis does not require a long period of time in which to induce a hypnotic trance. Indeed, with a skilled practitioner and an intelligent, motivated patient, induction can usually be accomplished very rapidly.

Other common misconceptions about hypnosis are discussed in the following section.

Common Misconceptions   In the popular imagination, the term "hypnosis" calls up images of the stage show hypnotist whose subjects are, like robots, compelled to carry out his every command. This view of hypnosis—the idea of a helpless subject and an all-powerful hypnotist—has never had the support of the scientific community. Unfortunately, the use of hypnosis for entertainment has given rise to a number of such misconceptions about its nature. Let us examine some of these myths.

Myth: Only weak-minded people can be hypnotized.

Comment: Hypnosis requires at least a degree of motivation and imagination. Thus, in general, intelligent individuals make better hypnotic subjects than mentally dull individuals. While it is almost certainly true that some people are more susceptible than others, one group of experts estimates that only about five percent of normal adults do not seem able to go into at least a light trance.

Myth: The hypnotized subject can be compelled to do things, even against his will.

Comment: While opinions vary somewhat as to how directive and authoritarian the professional using hypnosis should be with a patient in hypnosis, experts agree that it is the patient's trance. The patient decides whether or not he will cooperate with anything suggested to him. The patient does not lose control; in fact, in a trance state, the patient is able to control behaviors and functions that are normally not under voluntary control, such as salivation and blood flow.

Myth: Going into a trance can be dangerous because you might not be able to come out of it.

Comment: Since the patient retains ultimate control of his trance, it follows that he can terminate it whenever he wishes. If an emergency situation were to occur, such as a fire, the patient would come out of the trance immediately.

Fostering such misconceptions about the nature of hypnosis has probably retarded the acceptance of hypnosis as a legitimate therapeutic tool. For this reason at least, the use of hypnosis as entertainment is unacceptable. In fact, committees appointed by the British Medical Association and the American Medical Association to study hypnosis have, respectively, "deplored" and "condemned" the use of hypnosis for this purpose.[28]

What is Hypnosis?   What is hypnosis? How does it work? At present, there seems to be no scientifically acceptable definition of hypnosis. Some argue that hypnosis is truly an altered state of consciousness, a state quite different from our normal waking state of awareness; others disagree.* There is, however, general agreement on the following points.

- Hypnosis is a means of focusing the patient's attention and concentration.
- The person in hypnosis shows increased receptivity and readiness to respond to suggestion.
- The therapeutic effectiveness of hypnosis depends to a great extent on a good professional–patient relationship.

---

* *The author believes that there is sufficient evidence to consider deep trance, at least, as an altered state of consciousness.*

According to Dr. Milton Erikson, a psychiatrist who is widely known for his creative and imaginative use of hypnosis, hypnosis is used for the purpose of:

> . . . securing and fixating the patient's attention, creating in him a receptive and responsive mental state . . . to induce a favorable setting in which to instruct the patient in a more advantageous use of his own potentials of behavior.[29]

Each of us, Erikson would argue, has untapped skills and abilities which we do not even know we possess. In addition, each of us has a vast store of memories of past experiences, sounds, sights, and sensations. With the help of a skilled clinician, hypnosis allows us to tap and utilize these abilities and memories for our own benefit. Clinicians who make use of hypnosis stress that teaching a patient to enter a trance (trance induction) is rather simple; much greater skill is required in selecting and phrasing the suggestions, instructions, and ideas that will be of greatest benefit to the individual patient.

Research Findings As we noted earlier, the documented use of hypnosis to relieve pain associated with medical and dental surgery goes back well over a century. Since then, hypnosis has also been used, with sometimes dramatic success, to relieve pain associated with a variety of conditions, including childbirth, severe burns, and terminal illness.

The body of clinical evidence concerning the effectiveness of hypnosis in relieving pain is very large and quite compelling. Concerning research evidence, however, there is disagreement among experts. While one authority on chronic pain flatly asserts, "None of the reports I have been able to find are worth citing,"[30] another, equally well-known investigator states, "Pain reduction through hypnotic suggestion is demonstrated by all of those who have tried it, including the most skeptical."[31]

Some have suggested that the effects of hypnosis are really no different from placebo effects, as both involve strong suggestion, manipulation of attention and expectation, and reduction of anxiety. However, results of a well-controlled study show clearly that, in highly susceptible subjects, pain relief from hypnosis is distinct from that produced by placebo alone.[32]

Chaves and Barber[33] have argued that surgery under hypnosis is painless because most deep organs and tissues contain few pain receptors. However, Kay Thompson, a dentist who has lectured and written widely on the use of hypnosis, has produced a film of a patient undergoing dermabrasion with hypnosis as the only means of pain control. As dermabrasion is performed directly on the skin, where most of the pain receptors are located, this evidence would appear to invalidate Chaves and Barber's hypothesis.

Certainly, clear and compelling experimental evidence of hypnotic analgesia has been difficult to obtain, in large part because pain is such a private, subjective experience. When the event is one which can be more precisely and objectively measured, however, such as blood loss during surgery, the evidence is irrefutable: hypnosis results in significant reductions in blood loss during the operative and postoperative periods.[34]

We think that such evidence, together with the body of clinical data indicating the effectiveness of hypnosis in relieving pain, strongly supports the usefulness of this technique, and we urge dentists to add this skill to their repertories. Hypnosis is a noninvasive procedure and the dentist risks little in using it as a matter of routine. At worst, nothing will happen; at best, the effects may be extremely gratifying to dentist and patient alike.

CHRONIC PAIN CONDITIONS

Chronic pain is usually defined as pain which has persisted for six months or longer. Although we can distinguish between chronic pain which is malignant in origin, resulting from a life-threatening condition, and that which is benign or not life threatening, we should not interpret the term "benign" to mean "harmless." Chronic pain, no matter what the origin, usually results in profound disruption in the individual's life and can even lead to suicide.

Chronic pain differs from acute pain not only in duration but in other important aspects as well. Acute pain is situational, locatable, and specific. The patient in acute pain can look forward to a time when his pain will diminish. Chronic pain, on the other hand, is overwhelming and exhausting. The person who has suffered long, weary months or years of pain feels helpless. After trying numerous treatments and remedies to no avail, he may be bitter, angry and without hope.

Chronic Pain and Depression

From this description of chronic pain, we might expect to find that chronic pain patients are often depressed, and in fact, it is the very rare chronic pain patient who is not depressed. Just as anxiety is associated with acute pain, depression has been found to be closely related to chronic pain. In some cases, the experience of unremitting pain leads to depression; among other patients, a depressive episode may precipitate pain. It is also not uncommon to see patients in whom pain serves to "mask" or "stand for" an underlying depression. Under stress, instead of experiencing the subjective symptoms of depression, the patient experiences pain.

Pain may indicate depression if it is associated with physiological signs of depression, such as sleep disturbance and change in diurnal rhythms, or if a preexisting medical or dental condition worsens. If the pain is somewhat vague and nonspecific and difficult for the patient to describe or localize, the dentist should think of depression.

Richard Sternbach, a psychologist who has worked extensively with chronic pain patients, suggests that the relationship between pain and depression may reflect similar neurochemical processes underlying the two conditions.[30] This would account for the fact that many chronic pain patients obtain relief when given antidepressant medication.

Pain Transactions

Pain of long duration almost always leads to major changes in the patient's economic, interpersonal, and emotional functioning. The boundaries of the patient's life constrict and his world comes to center around his pain. Others begin to take over his responsibilities, and activities from which he previously derived satisfaction, self-esteem, and recognition from others are abandoned. At the same time, he may receive considerable sympathy and attention from those around him when he evidences pain.

More and more, then, the patient views himself in terms of his pain, and his pain becomes the means by which he communicates with and relates to others. His identity becomes that of a person who is in pain.

This notion has important implications for the health care professional because—although such a patient is usually completely unaware of his own manipulative attempts—his interaction with health care professionals often takes the form of efforts designed to maintain his identity. These efforts, which Sternbach has termed "pain games," result in patient and professional working at cross purposes. The patient, to preserve his identity, needs to keep his pain; the professional, to confirm his own identity, must try to relieve the pain. If the professional becomes too caught up in the challenge of succeeding where numerous others have failed or believes that he must cure or relieve all pain in order to consider himself a "success," he can easily become trapped in a "game," with much frustration as the result.

Management of Chronic Pain Conditions

Although the chronic pain conditions the dentist in general practice is likely to see are relatively few in number (trigeminal neuralgia and mysofascial pain dysfunction syndrome are the most common), the diagnosis of a facial pain can sometimes be a difficult and challenging task. Part of the problem is that facial pain can have its origin in many different organs and structures.

Patients, however, seldom realize this and understandably assume that a pain in the oral region indicates a dental disorder. The dentist, of course, must be quite cautious in accepting the patient's diagnosis of the problem. In an informative article on the diagnosis of orofacial pain, the author points out:

The dentist must remember that because a patient has sought his help does not necessarily mean that the patient has a dental problem . . . If the dentist accepts the patient's diagnosis of a dental problem without question, he may well overlook the real cause of the pain and provide unnecessary dental treatment.[35]

As an example of a condition in which unnecessary dental treatment has all too often been provided, the author cites trigeminal neuralgia and quotes from a review of over 270 patients with this disorder:

The prime reason why trigeminal neuralgia must be recognized at an early stage is to avoid unnecessary dental treatment; almost every case presented having had partial or complete extractions . . . Never in the history of dentistry has so much been done to so many with so little benefit.

For this reason, the dentist should never perform irreversible procedures unless he is absolutely sure of the diagnosis. When there exists any doubt, the patient should be referred to the appropriate specialist for evaluation. Obviously, the more the dentist knows about the origins and differential diagnoses of facial pain, the more likely it becomes that he will be able to refer the patient appropriately.

In some cases, especially if the patient has already made the rounds of numerous specialists, a referral to a pain clinic or center is warranted. These clinics, which have proliferated across the county, are staffed by multidisciplinary teams trained to provide a variety of diagnostic and treatment approaches to the problem of chronic pain. A list of more than 300 such clinics across the country can be obtained, for a small fee, by writing to: The American Society of Anesthesiologists, 515 Busse Highway, Park Ridge, Illinois 60068.

REFERENCES

1. Weisenberg, M. *Pain: Clinical and Experimental Perspectives*. St. Louis: C. V. Mosby, 1975, p. 259.
2. Beecher, H. K. "Quantification of the subjective pain experience." In *Psychopathology of Perception,* edited by P. H. Hoch and J. Zubin. New York: Grune and Stratton, 1965.
3. Melzack, R. *The Puzzle of Pain.* New York: Basic Books, 1973.
4. Melzack, R. and Wall, P. D. "Pain mechanisms: A new theory." *Science* 150:971, 1965.

5. Merskey, H. and Spear, E. H. *Pain: Psychological and Psychiatric Aspects*. London: Bailliere, Tindall and Cassell, 1967.

6. Melzack, R. and Scott, T. H. "The effects of early experience on the response to pain." *J Comp Physiol Psychol* 50:155, 1957.

7. Hardy, J. D.; Wolff, G. H.; Goodell, H. *Pain Sensations and Reactions*. New York: Hafner, 1952.

8. Sternbach, R. A. and Tursky, B. "Ethnic differences among housewives in psychophysical and skin potential responses to electric shock." *Psychophysiology* 1:241, 1965.

9. Fordyce, W. E. *Behavioral Methods for Chronic Pain and Illness*. St. Louis: C. V. Mosby, 1976.

10. Loan, W. B. and Morrison, J. D. "The incidence and severity of postoperative pain." *Brit J Anesth* 39:695, 1967.

11. Pilowsky, I. and Bond, M. R. "Pain and its management in malignant disease: Elucidation of staff–patient transactions. *Psychosomatic Med* 31:400, 1969.

12. Hill, H. E.; Kornetsky, C. H.; Flanary, H. G.; Wikler, A. "Studies on anxiety associated with anticipation of pain: I. Effects of morphine." *Arch Neur Psychiat* 67:612, 1952.

13. Kanfer, F. H. and Godlfoot, D. A. "Self-control and tolerance of noxious stimulation." *Psycholog Reports* 18:79, 1966.

14. Barber, T. X. and Cooper, B. J. "Effects on pain of experimentally induced and spontaneous distraction." *Psycholog Reports* 24:647, 1972.

15. Gardner, W. J. and Licklider, J. C. R. "Auditory analgesia in dental operations." *Am Dent A J* 59:1144, 1959.

16. Klepac, R. K. "The role of pain in dental apprehension." In *Clinical Research in Behavioral Dentistry: Proceedings of the Second National Conference on Behavioral Dentistry*, edited by B. D. Ingersoll and W. R. McCutcheon, pp. 52–63. Morgantown, W. Va.: West Virginia University, 1979.

17. Egbert, L. D.; Battit, G. E.; Welch, C. E.; Bartlett, M. K. "Reduction of post-operative pain by encouragement and instruction of patients." *N E J Med* 270:825, 1964.

18. Evans, F. J. "Placebo analgesia: Suggestion, anxiety, and the doctor–patient relationship." Paper presented at the meeting of the American Psychosomatic Society, Philadelphia, March, 1974.

19. Beecher, H. K. "Relationship of significance of wound to the pain experienced." *Am Med A J* 161:1609, 1956.

20. Bobey, M. J. and Davidson, P. O. "Psychological factors affecting pain tolerance." *J Psychosomt Res* 14:371, 1970.

21. Gessel, A. H. and Alderman, M. M. "Management of myofascial pain dysfunction syndrome of the temporomandibular joint by tension control training." *Psychosomatics* 12:302, 1971.

22. Wolf, S. "Effects of suggestion and conditioning on the action of chemical agents in human subjects." *J Clin Invest* 29:100, 1950.

23. Laskin, D. M. and Greene, C. S. "Influence of the doctor–patient relationship on placebo therapy for patients with myofascial pain dysfunction (MPD) syndrome. *Am Dent A J* 85:892, 1972.

24. Beecher, H. K. *Measurement of Subjective Responses: Quantitative Effects of Drugs.* New York: Oxford University Press, 1959.
25. Beecher, H. K. "Increased stress and effectiveness of placebos and 'active' drugs." *Science* 132:91, 1960.
26. Gryll, S. L. and Katahn, M. "Situational factors contributing to the placebo effect." *Psychopharm* 57:253, 1978.
27. Hass, H.; Fink, H.; Harfelder, G. "Das Placeboproblem." *Fortschr Arzneimittel forschung,* 1:279, 1959. Translation of selected parts in *Psychopharm Ser Ctr Bul* 2:1, 1963.
28. American Society of Clinical Hypnosis, Education, and Research Foundation. *A Syllabus on Hypnosis and a Handbook of Therapeutic Suggestions.* Des Plaines, Illinois, 1973.
29. Erikson, M. H. "The interspersal hypnotic technique for sympton correction and pain control." *Clin Hypnosis A J* 8:198, 1966.
30. Sternbach, R. A. *Pain Patients: Traits and Treatment.* New York: Academic Press, 1974.
31. Hilgard, E. R. "A neodissociation interpretation of pain reduction in hypnosis." *Psychol Rev* 80:396, 1973.
32. McGlashan, T. H.; Evans, F. J.; Orne, M. T. "The nature of hypnotic analgesia and placebo response to experimental pain." *Psychosomt Med* 31:227, 1969.
33. Chaves, J. F. and Barber, T. X. "Hypnotism and surgical pain." In *Hypnosis, Imagination and Human Potentialities,* edited by T. X. Barber, N. P. Spanos, and J. F. Chaves. New York: Pergamon Press, 1974.
34. Chaves, J. F.; Wilden, D.; Roller, N. "Hypnosis in dental behavioral science: Control of surgical and post-surgical bleeding." In *Clinical Research in Behavioral Dentistry: Proceedings of the Second National Conference on Behavioral Dentistry,* edited by B. D. Ingersoll and W. R. McCutcheon, pp. 95–107. Morgantown, W. Va.: West Virginia University, 1979.
35. Drinnan, A. J. "Differential diagnosis of orofacial pain." *Dent Clin N Am* 22:73–87, 1978.

6

Motivation, Compliance, and Preventive Behavior

Patients who do not follow health care recommendations are encountered by all health care professionals. In a recent comprehensive review, it was reported that between 30 percent and 70 percent of all recommendations for medication, home care, exercise, diet, and the like were not followed by patients.[1]

It should come as no surprise that dentists encounter their full share of such patients and results of recent surveys indicate that these problems are widespread, indeed. In a national survey of practicing dentists, three-quarters of the dentists surveyed cited "patients not following treatment instructions" as a problem in their practices.[2] Orthodontists and prosthodontists are especially troubled by such patients; over half of these specialists in the sample surveyed reported the problem. We can speculate that this may be due, at least in part, to the fact that treatment instructions in these specialities are often somewhat complicated and require that the patient make special efforts to follow them.

Results of this same survey also highlighted problems in patient compliance with preventive recommendations. Over two-thirds of the dentists surveyed complained of "patients who seem ignorant of the benefits of preventive care"—that is, patients who seek emergency care only, demand extractions when restorative procedures could be performed, and the like. Younger dentists (those in practice for less than ten years) emerged as the group most likely to cite this problem. With the recent heavy emphasis on prevention in dental education in recent years, it is not surprising that young practitioners would consider preventive care important and feel special concern over problems in this area.

Finally, as is well known, dentists frequently complain of "patients who do not seem well motivated to engage in good home care practices." Three-quarters of the dentists surveyed reported this problem, with orthodontists, periodontists, and prosthodontists citing it with special frequency.

These findings will come as no surprise to the dentist or dental student. What is, perhaps, surprising—and certainly disheartening—is the frequency with which the dentist encounters noncompliant patients. One researcher studying patient compliance with recommendations for professional preventive care and home care reported that, of the patients he studied, only about one-third were highly compliant, about half were moderately compliant, and about one-fourth were considered noncompliant.[3]

This means that, under ordinary conditions, only about three out of every ten patients you see will follow your preventive recommendations and meet your expectations. The remainder will disregard some or all of your recommendations.

What, if anything, can be done to alter the behavior of such patients? In this section, we will discuss the question, examine research evidence related to the issue, and suggest some methods for obtaining improved rates of compliance from your patients.

BELIEF SYSTEMS AND COMPLIANCE: THE HEALTH CARE BELIEF MODEL

What is known about the differences between patients who comply with preventive recommendations and those who do not? Many authors have stated that personality differences distinguish compliant patients from noncompliant patients. Some have suggested, for example, that the noncompliant patient has passive–aggressive traits or that he has trouble with authority figures. However, research has failed to support these notions or the more general concept of personality differences between the two groups.

The only consistent difference between the groups that has emerged from the results of several studies is a difference in the health belief systems of each group. Specifically, we find that people who engage in preventive activities believe that:

- they are vulnerable to a specific disease
- the disease could have serious consequences
- by engaging in preventive activities, they can reduce the likelihood or seriousness of the disease.[4]

These beliefs are held to a much lesser extent by individuals who do not regularly engage in preventive activities.

This, then, is the basis of the Health Care Belief Model which has received so much attention in the medical and dental literature in recent years. The essential points of the model are, as noted above, that people will engage in preventive activities and comply with medical and dental recommendations only if they believe that they are susceptible to a serious disease and, further, that their own actions will influence the probability that they will actually contract the disease.

How helpful is such knowledge to the dentist who attempts to promote better compliance among his patients? Is the Health Care Belief Model useful in suggesting strategies to improve compliance? Unfortunately, the model provides little useful information for the practicing dentist.

The model itself is essentially a descriptive model only. That is, we know that there is a relationship between health care beliefs and health care behavior, but we cannot demonstrate that certain beliefs cause certain behaviors.

Many researchers (and many more individual practitioners) have assumed such a causative relationship between beliefs and behavior and directed their energies toward changing beliefs in the hope that behavior change will follow. Educational programs—many of them quite massive in scope—have, in fact, been the most common approach to improving preventive behavior. Certainly, the educational approach has intuitive appeal. It is comforting to think that people are rational creatures who would do what is good for them if only they had the appropriate information.

Unfortunately, however, we know that this is not the case. Study after study has shown that educational efforts to encourage better oral health care behavior have achieved little success. Taken together, the results of numerous educational programs designed to teach the public the facts about dental disease and the need for preventive activities are disappointing. These results show that educational programs:

- can produce impressive increases in knowledge about dental disease and appropriate preventive activities
- can result in marked changes in attitudes toward dental health
- can produce short-term improvement in preventive behavior
- do not produce long-term improvement in preventive behavior.

The prevention of oral disease requires significant alterations in patient behavior over very lengthy periods—indeed, over an entire lifetime. The evidence is clear: educational programs alone do not produce such changes.

The failure of educational/informational programs to produce significant long-term improvement in preventive behavior led some investigators to try fear appeals. This approach, which some believed would have a greater impact than simple information, was essentially an attempt to scare people into engaging in preventive activities. Research showed, however, that the use of fear messages was not an effective means of producing change. If the level of fear contained in the message was very high (i.e., showing gory pictures of patients with advanced oral diseases), people simply "tuned out" the entire message. Messages which employed moderate or low levels of fear led to no greater improvement in preventive behavior than that obtained with simple informational approaches.

Does this mean that providing information about preventive behavior is of no value whatsoever? We do not mean to imply that this is the case. Certainly, patients need to know the facts about their own vulnerability to oral disease, and they need specific information about exactly what preventive activities are required and how often these activities must be carried out.

In general, dentists appear to be doing a good job of providing patients with such information. As Dr. Philip Weinstein, writer and researcher in prevention, has noted:

> I have found that many dental offices routinely provide more than enough information concerning the etiology, histopathology, and sequelae of dental disease. Patients usually are provided with the necessary data to choose health-related goals.[5]

However, he states, "The instruction they need to achieve these goals is rarely made available. To achieve these goals," he continues, "patients need skill training, and they require assistance in developing new habit patterns —in short, they need help in changing their behavior."

In summary, while information can provide initial motivation through changing a patient's beliefs and attitudes, our ultimate goal must be to change the patient's behavior. Strategies for implementing behavior change are discussed in the following sections.

PRODUCING BEHAVIOR CHANGE

Everyone who has ever tried to change his own behavior—tried to break an old habit pattern or begin a new one—knows that producing long-term changes in behavior is not an easy task. Several factors influence the ease or difficulty with which behavior change can be produced. In general, we find that it is more difficult to produce behavior change if:

- the behavior requires the individual to assume an active, continuous role
- the behavior is difficult, intrusive, or time consuming
- the consequences of the behavior are long range and/or uncertain.

The Patient's Role

It is more difficult to produce behavior change if the behavior requires the individual to assume an active, continuous role. Preventive activities can be placed along a continuum of active-vs-passive patient role and along a continuum of frequency, from single events to activities which must be performed on an ongoing, or continuous, basis. Most people are willing to engage in one-shot preventive activities which allow them to play a rather passive role, such as receiving an inoculation to prevent contagious disease. Unfortunately, we do not have a procedure comparable to the inoculation available at this time in dentistry.

Toward the middle of the active–passive continuum and the frequency continuum are preventive recommendations which require periodic visits to professionals for routine preventive care, cleaning, and such technical procedures as topical fluoride treatments and occlusal surface sealants. People are often willing to comply with recommendations for these procedures. In fact, research shows that, in general, people are more likely to comply with recommendations for preventive activities which involve clinic care than with those which involve self-care.[3,6]

Of course, this does not mean that you will be successful in persuading all of your patients to complete a course of treatment or come in for regular checkups and prophylaxis. We are all familiar with the patient who, encouraged to make a return appointment before leaving the office, mumbles, "I'll call you." True to his word, he calls—two years later and in pain!

Even if you are successful in persuading patients to make return appointments before leaving the office, you have no guarantee that they will actually keep these appointments. Broken or cancelled appointments are a too familiar fact of life to most dentists. As we noted earlier, three-quarters of dentists recently surveyed complained of this problem. Broken appointment rates are generally reported to be more than 20 percent and can run as high as 50 percent.[7]

Several strategies have been suggested to help remedy this situation. The most commonly used are the reminder note and the reminder telephone call. How well do these methods work to reduce the rate of broken or cancelled appointments?

In a study undertaken in a clinic with a 30 percent broken appointment rate, telephone reminders decreased the rate to 24 percent and post-card reminders decreased the rate to 21 percent.[8] The ineffectiveness of the telephone reminder was linked to difficulty in contacting patients by telephone to remind them of the impending appointment—a difficulty typically encountered with the telephone reminder strategy. (It should also be noted that this method is costly in terms of staff time, a further disadvantage.)

The most successful method was found to be asking the patient to call the clinic to confirm his appointment. The receptionist gave each patient a reminder card which contained instructions for calling to confirm. She also asked the patient to call, implying that she was the person to whom the patient would be speaking. This provided a more personal touch than simply a written request on the card. This method reduced the broken appointment rate to 12 percent, a significant drop from the baseline rate of 30 percent.

An additional point worth noting is that almost all (98 percent) of the patients in this group who did call to confirm their appointments kept them; the broken appointments were almost exclusively in the group that did not call to confirm. This suggests that the most cost-effective strategy for reducing broken appointments is to request all patients to call to confirm their appointments. For those who fail to confirm by the designated time, a telephone reminder call can be made the day before the appointment.

The Nature of the Behavior

It is more difficult to produce behavior change if the behavior is difficult, intrusive, or time consuming. Again, we find that home care procedures fall in the difficult range. A good home care program is time consuming. It has been estimated that a thorough plaque-control regimen carried out once a day with one or two additional brushings can take as long as 30 minutes per day. If we assume a waking day of 16 hours, we find that three percent of the patient's waking time is devoted to oral hygiene.

Home care procedures are also intrusive. They compete with other activities the patient finds more pressing or more enjoyable. Bad timing may be one factor contributing to the problem. Most people brush and floss just before going to bed. However, after we've completed a round of prebedtime chores which can include making lunches and setting out clothes for the next day, locking the house, setting the thermostat, letting the cat out, and checking on the kids, few of us are in the mood to do a thorough job of brushing and flossing, unless the habit is very deeply ingrained.

For patients who are attempting to acquire good oral hygiene habits, such poor timing can be a major stumbling block. These patients may need help in improving the timing of their home care regimen. For example, you can suggest to a patient who always watches the late news that he brush and floss before the news—or even while watching the news. In this way, watching the news can serve as a reward for brushing and flossing, thereby strengthening the habit. (We will discuss the importance of rewards in the following section.)

Finally, while we are reluctant to describe brushing and flossing as "difficult," they are behaviors which require a certain amount of skill if they are to be performed effectively. A word of caution: do not assume that your patients know how to brush and floss properly; ask them to demonstrate their technique for you. If you find that their skills are deficient, a training program is necessary.

A good program to teach motor skills such as brushing and flossing includes each of the following:

1. *Demonstration.* People learn most efficiently when they are shown what to do, rather than simply told. A variety of film strips and videotapes demonstrating the correct brushing and flossing techniques are readily available. If you own home video equipment, you and your assistants can easily make your own teaching tapes.

2. *Practice with feedback.* Feedback about the accuracy of one's performance is essential to good motor skills learning. At each office visit, the patient should be given specific information about the adequacy of his efforts. The more specific the feedback the better. A number of oral hygiene indices have been developed which yield numerical scores and, although use of such scales requires additional time and effort, a numerical score is preferable to a vague "You're doing better," or "You need to improve," especially for the patient who has room for improvement. Graphing the patient's score at each visit so he can view his progress (or lack thereof) can be especially helpful. Even greater visual impact can be achieved with a simple color-coded graph in which a band of one color covers scores in the "poor" range, a second color represents the "fair" range, and a third color represents the "good" range. Using such graphs in our own clinic, we have obtained promising results in improved parental care of their young children's teeth.

The immediacy of feedback is also important. Without the immediate (and unpleasant) auditory feedback of grinding machinery to inform the novice driver that he has not shifted gears properly, few transmissions would survive the beginner's attempts. What cues might be used as immediate feedback to inform the patient of the adequacy of his brushing and flossing? Most, if not all, adult patients can discriminate between the taste of a clean mouth and one which has not been adequately cleaned, so these sensations might serve as feedback. Unfortunately, however, flavored toothpastes provide the taste of a clean mouth, even when the patient has not brushed and flossed adequately. To eliminate this problem, Dr. James Cassidy, a prominent dental educator, suggests that patients be taught to brush with a dry brush initially. When they can achieve the taste and sensation of a clean mouth using only a dry brush and floss, they have mastered brushing and flossing skills and can return to using toothpaste.

Although many dentists delegate responsibility for teaching oral hygiene skills to their auxiliaries, remember that, as a dentist, you retain responsibility for the work of your employees. Remember, too, that patient compliance with recommendations is related to the status of the person who makes the recommendations. One study,[9] for example, demonstrated that patient compliance with recommendations made by a dentist was significantly better than compliance when the same recommendation was made by a dental assistant. It is important that you lend your prestige to back up the significance of what is taught by your auxiliaries.

The Use of Consequences to Change Behavior

It is more difficult to produce behavior change if the consequences are long range and/or uncertain. The consequences which follow a behavior play an important role in learning. Behavior is affected most strongly by consequences which immediately follow the behavior. When there is a delay between a behavior (for example overeating) and the consequences which follow (weight gain), the consequences are not likely to have a marked effect on the behavior.

In general, negative or aversive consequences following a behavior serve to weaken the behavior, decreasing the probability that it will occur again. If you put your hand on a hot stove and suffer a painful burn (negative consequences) as a result, you will be less likely to touch hot stoves in the future.

On the other hand, positive or rewarding consequences following a behavior serve to strengthen the behavior. Positive consequences increase the likelihood that the behavior will be repeated. Behavior change is facilitated if events are arranged so that consequences are positive, immediate, and certain.

Parents, teachers, and animal trainers have often made good, if unsystematic, use of these principles. Recently, following the lead of Harvard psychologist B. F. Skinner, who pioneered reinforcement (reward) theory, psychologists have systematically and successfully applied these principles to a very broad range of human behavior. We can draw upon their work to help our patients learn better oral health behaviors.

Selection and Use of Positive Consequences Consequences need not be dramatic in order to alter behavior, nor are they always immediately apparent to an observer. A smile can serve as a powerful reward; a frown can serve as an effective punishing agent. Although most of us immediately think of material goods at the mention of the word "reward," there are other types of positive consequences which can serve as well, or even better, to strengthen behavior.

- *Social rewards* include attention, smiles, winks, hugs, praise, and other signs of approval and affection. We often underestimate the power of social rewards, but they can be surprisingly effective in producing behavior change.
- *Activity rewards* include any activity a person enjoys, such as watching television, going to a party, reading a book, or playing a game. Activity rewards need not be special events. Any activity which the person enjoys or performs regularly can be used to reward any other behavior. Thus, T.V. time, making a phone call, or even taking a bath could be very useful activity rewards for some people.
- *Material rewards* include any material item a person can use, wear, play

with, or consume. Money, toys, food, and clothing are all material rewards. Material rewards can be very effective in promoting behavior change, but programs which rely only on material rewards can quickly become quite expensive.

Of course, what is rewarding to one individual might not be rewarding to another; in fact, it might even be punishing. In order to be effective, a reward must be truly rewarding to the person who receives it.

We have stressed the need for positive consequences to occur immediately following a desired behavior. This is not always possible, especially when the reward is a baseball game or a movie. Point programs are useful under these circumstances: the individual earns a point each time he performs the behavior and a certain number of points is required to earn the reward.

An additional advantage of a point program is that it provides a good method for collecting data on the behavior in question. Keeping written records of behavior is very important when you are attempting to produce behavior change. Human memory is notoriously unreliable and most people, relying only on memory, tend to overestimate or underestimate in their favor.

Records not only allow the person to monitor his progress accurately, but they also can, themselves, serve as positive consequences as the person sees how much he has accomplished. Sometimes, in fact, no additional consequences are necessary to produce an initial change in behavior; the simple act of recording each instance of brushing and flossing is often sufficient to produce improvement in these behaviors. This is especially likely to occur if the patient is provided with "official" self-monitoring forms and is instructed to bring the completed forms to his next appointment (which should be scheduled within two weeks or so). Although self-monitoring effects usually tend to be somewhat short-lived, and thus should be supplemented with additional measures, they can be very beneficial in getting the patient off to a good start.

So far, we have directed attention only to rewards which are externally administered. Rewards can also be self-administered. In fact, for most of us, self-administered rewards, such as telling ourselves "That's a good job," or "I'm a hard worker," probably play an essential role in maintaining many of our everyday behaviors. People can be taught to employ reward programs to effectively manage their own behavior without external intervention. Instructions for implementing such programs, as well as many good examples, can be found in Weinstein and Getz's useful book, *Changing Human Behavior: Strategies for Preventive Dentistry.* *

---

* *Chicago: SRA, 1978.*

Using Positive Consequences with Child Patients What rewards can the dentist provide for good oral hygiene behavior? The dentist who has a good relationship with his child patients can use social rewards with good results. In addition, he can use a variety of other rewards for lowered plaque scores. Examples include prizes, trophies, wallet cards, and club memberships. Children can be encouraged to keep daily records of brushing and flossing and to bring these records with them to the appointment.

A word of caution: especially when working with children, it is important to set reasonable and realistic goals and to provide rewards for small steps toward improvement. The dentist who waits until his patient's plaque score is almost perfect before rewarding the patient may never see his patients reach their goals. It is much more effective to ask for incremental changes, one step at a time.

Although you can provide some consequences for good home care practices, your effectiveness is limited by your infrequent contact with the child. Therefore, you can probably be most effective in promoting proper home care behaviors if you teach parents to set up reward programs in the home. Parents can be taught to use this approach effectively. One investigator found that children whose parents had been taught to reward them for brushing and flossing had much better oral health, as indicated by plaque and gingival measures, than children in a control group.[10]

When instructing parents in the use of reward programs for their children, keep the following points in mind.

• Provide parents with charts on which points (or stars, for younger children) can be entered for daily performance.
• Help parents avoid the material reward trap. Encourage them to make use of social rewards and activity rewards. Activity rewards can be inexpensive, easy to use, and very effective with children. (One investigator, using swimming as a reward for toothbrushing in a summer camp for boys, increased the rate of daily brushing from about zero to almost 100 percent![11]) Among the activity rewards that children especially enjoy are late bedtimes, having a friend stay over, and dinner at McDonald's.
• Urge parents to provide rewards frequently, especially when the child is first learning the new habits. We have had considerable success with a "double-barrel" approach which permits the child to earn a small daily reward, such as a bedtime story, and to accumulate points toward a larger reward, such as a bowling trip or having a friend stay over.
• Involve the child in choosing rewards. Occasionally, a child will request a reward that the family considers inappropriate or too expensive. Initially the child may refuse attempts at negotiation, insisting that, if he cannot have a dog (or a horse or a mini-bike), he doesn't want anything at all. The wise parent will not argue. Instead, he will drop the subject and simply arrange other, more appropriate rewards which he knows the child

enjoys. The child might hold out for a day or two, but if the rewards are carefully selected, he will usually decide to "get with the program."

Parents are usually willing to implement reward programs such as those we have described. However, they often have questions about the programs. Below are some of the more common questions we have encountered.

Q. Aren't rewards really bribes?

A: Rewards are not bribes. The dictionary defines a bribe as "Anything given to induce a person to do something illegal or wrong." There is nothing illegal or wrong about oral hygiene behavior.

Q: Why should a child be rewarded for something he should be doing anyway?

A: If a child is to learn to do things we think he should do, rewards can facilitate learning. Remember, it is not necessary to use material rewards; the child can earn some of his privileges as rewards for good behavior.

Q: How long must I continue to use a reward program?

A: Continue to use a reward program until the new behavior is well established (usually a period of several weeks to a few months). Then rewards can be faded out gradually. One approach is to tell the child that no longer will every performance of the behavior be rewarded; that, instead, surprise spot checks will be made. If he has performed the behavior, he will earn a reward; if not, no reward. Initially, spot checks should be made every other day or so, then decreased to every three to four days and so on until they are no longer necessary. If the child begins to backslide, reinstitute the reward program temporarily. Eventually, the results of the behavior (sensation of a clean mouth) will become rewarding to the child and the habit will be firmly established.

Using Positive Consequences with Adult Patients Employing positive consequences with adult patients poses a different set of problems from those encountered in developing reward programs for child patients. It also requires more ingenuity on the part of the dentist.

Although children may have little real concern about or desire to improve their oral hygiene, they are brought to the dentist by their parents, who indicate at least some degree of interest in their child's oral health by the very fact that they have made and kept an appointment for the child. Thus, it is usually not too difficult to enlist the parents' aid in helping the child learn good oral health behavior.

Obviously the situation with the adult patient is quite different. Unlike the child patient, the adult patient himself must make a decision to alter his behavior and, once having made this decision, he must also serve as his own principal source of positive consequences.

Sometimes, of course, patients do not have any desire to improve their oral hygiene practices, despite your best attempts to educate and motivate them. What can you do in this situation? Weinstein discusses this situation in terms of problem ownership. The dentist, he says, must decide whether the patient's poor oral hygiene is the patient's problem (does it bother the patient?) or the professional's problem (is the professional the only one who is bothered by the situation?). He offers some useful guidelines for communicating with such patients but concludes that, with some patients, the dentist might have to lower his own expectations.

Some practitioners feel differently. "Why," they argue, "should I waste my time and skill on a patient who doesn't care enough to do his part?" We believe that this is a defensible point of view. Further, we think that it is legitimate for the dentist to place certain demands on his patients and to specify the conditions under which he will agree to provide treatment. Dr. Robert Bricker, past president of the West Virginia Dental Association, does just that. He makes a contractual agreement with each new patient at the first visit. According to the contract, Dr. Bricker will begin treatment only when the patient has reached a certain level of oral hygiene. It is the rare patient, Dr. Bricker reports, who fails to live up to the contract.

Contracts which employ positive consequences can also be based on your professional fees. A sliding fee scale, with higher fees for noncompliant patients, rewards the compliant patient for good home care. People are often more willing to make changes when those changes involve their pocketbook, as shown in a study[12] in which patients received fee reductions for improvements in oral hygiene. In this study, patients underwent a three-visit program of instruction in proper oral hygiene techniques. Patients who were then rewarded with a ten percent fee reduction for a plaque index of 20 percent or less and a fee reduction of 25 percent for a plaque index of ten percent or less achieved significantly lower plaque scores than patients who participated in the educational program but did not receive contingent fee reductions. This improvement was maintained at a six-month follow-up visit, an indication that this approach can have beneficial long-term effects.

When using contracts such as those we have described, remember to ask for gradual changes in the patient's behavior. Some dentists mistakenly believe that they should ask for a great deal of improvement initially in order to obtain even a small amount of change. This approach leads to discouragement and failure in the long run. As we noted previously, ask for change in small steps. Set reasonable goals and give the patient frequent appointments during the period in which he is establishing new habits.

Finally, do not underestimate the value of your own relationship with your patients. Your patients may value your opinion more than you realize. In fact, there have been studies which have shown that some patients avoid the dentist because they are afraid that he will criticize the condition of their mouths and belittle or scold them for this. This suggests that your enthusiasm, interest, and praise can serve to facilitate improvement in your patients' behavior.

REFERENCES

1. Sackett, D. and Haynes, R. *Compliance with Therapeutic Regimens.* Baltimore: Johns Hopkins University Press, 1976.
2. Ingersoll, B.; Ingersoll, T.; McCutcheon, W.; Seime, R. "Behavioral dimensions of dental practice: A national survey." West Virginia University School of Dentistry, 1979.
3. Davis, Unpublished manuscript, summarized in Bailit HL, 1978, personal communication.
4. Lund, A.; Kegles, S.; Weisenberg, M. "A children's dental program: Social psychology in public health dentistry." Paper presented at the meeting of the American Psychological Association, Washington, D.C., September, 1976.
5. Weinstein, P. "Behavioral strategies to enhance patient compliance with preventive recommendations." In *Advances in Behavioral Research in Dentistry,* edited by P. Weinstein. Seattle: University of Washington, 1978.
6. Lund, A. and Kegles, S. "Children's preventive dental programs." In *Behavioral Dentistry: Proceedings of the First National Conference,* edited by B. Ingersoll, R. Seime, W. McCutcheon. Morgantown, W. Va.: West Virginia University, 1977.
7. Sackett, D. "The magnitude of compliance and noncompliance." In *Compliance with Therapeutic Regimens,* edited by D. Sackett and R. Haynes. Baltimore: Johns Hopkins University Press, 1976.
8. Cohen, A. "Strategies to reduce broken dental appointments." In *Advances in Behavioral Research in Dentistry,* edited by P. Weinstein. Seattle: University of Washington, 1978.
9. Levine, B. A.; Moss, K. C.; Ramsey, P. H.; Fleishman, R. A. "Patient compliance with advice as a function of communicator expertise." *J Soc Psychol* 104:309, 1978.
10. Greenberg, J. "A study of behavior modification applied to dental health." *J Sch Health* 47:594, 1977.
11. Lattal, K. "Contingency management of toothbrushing behavior in a summer camp for children." *J Appl Behav Anal* 2:195, 1969.
12. Iwata, B. A. and Becksfort, C. M. "Behavioral research in preventive dentistry: Educational and contingency management approaches to the problem of patient compliance." *J Appl Behav Anal* 14:111, 1981.

7

Behavior Management in Pedodontics

The behavior of his child patients is of considerable importance to every dentist who treats children. The difficulties and risks of attempting to provide care to a child who is doing his physical and vocal best to protest can be so stressful that some dentists refuse to include children among their patients.

The child, as well as the dental staff, suffers as a result of such an experience. As McElroy[1] noted as long ago as 1895, "Although the operative dentistry may be perfect, the appointment is a failure if the child departs in tears." Virtually all writers on the subject agree that dental attitudes developed in childhood have great influence on later dental attitudes and behavior. Negative or traumatic early experiences can lead to fear and avoidance of dental care for long years after the child patient has become an adult.[2]

If we wish to prevent future avoidance of dental treatment, it is clear that we must do all we can to make the child's early dental visits as pleasant and enjoyable as possible. The realization of this goal demands more than good intentions; certain knowledge and skills are also necessary.

In this chapter, we will discuss factors which contribute to the child's reaction to the dental experience. We will also present a variety of approaches which have been used successfully to reduce fear and uncooperative behavior and to promote positive attitudes toward dentistry.

CHILDREN'S ATTITUDES TOWARD THE DENTAL EXPERIENCE

Several studies have attempted to answer the question, "How do children feel about visiting the dentist?" This question is actually more complex than it appears because there are many factors involved in a visit to the dentist. In general, however, while many children do admit to mild apprehension and a much smaller number intensely fear and dislike dental treatment, most grade school children and adolescents express attitudes which range from neutral to mildly positive toward the dental experience.[3,4] In fact, when children are asked, "What is the worst thing about going to the dentist?", a surprising number respond, "Nothing."

When asked, "What is the best thing about going to the dentist?", children commonly mention good dental care and prophylaxis. They are especially enthusiastic about the rewards or gifts dispensed by the dentist, as most clinicians have long known. This finding lends support to the idea that gifts promote positive feelings toward the dental visit and suggests that a gift should be given at the end of the visit, regardless of the child's behavior during the visit.

Attitudes Toward the Dentist

Personal liking for the dentist and his staff appears to play an especially important role in children's attitudes toward dentistry. In fact, the people working with the child are almost certainly more important than any other aspect of the dental experience, including aspects of the physical environment.

It is gratifying to note that, when asked how they feel about the dentist himself, most grade school children report positive feelings.[3,4] In fact, one group of researchers found that, although their fifth- and sixth-grade subjects did not rate "dentist" as highly as "father" on an evaluative scale, "dentist" was not rated differently from the concepts "doctor," "teacher," "friend," and "myself."[5] We can infer that the dentist–child relationship is one which is quite positive in the minds of many children.

The attitude of the parent is important, too, as it is the parent who selects the dentist, arranges the appointment, and ensures that instructions and recommendations are carried out. Among parents who are satisfied with their child's dentist, many cite "his relationship with children" as the reason for their satisfaction. Interestingly, although more parents—especially among the higher socioeconomic groups—cite "professional competence" as the reason, most parents are not really able to assess technical competence, as studies have clearly shown. As one author has suggested, parents may see the dentist's agreeable personal characteristics as evidence of his technical competence.[6]

The Physical Environment

It was not so long ago that dental operatories were visually negative places, with cord handpieces, cuspidors, and bracket trays with large collections of mysterious and frightening instruments all in full view of the child patient. The move toward streamlining the operatory and locating all equipment and instruments out of sight has produced operatories which are less clinical and intimidating in appearance.

There is little doubt that this trend has been beneficial for the child patient. Many children—especially females—express fear of the dental tools and instruments and the sight of the equipment appears to sensitize inexperienced children.[7] In one interesting study,[8] anxiety scores of dentally inexperienced children treated in a modified operatory (all apparatus kept out of sight) were lower than anxiety scores of children treated in an operatory with all equipment visible. Children were also less anxious if they were first interviewed in an interview room rather than in the operatory.

Bright colors are appealing to children, as are familiar cartoon characters and cheerful pictures and posters. It is probably wise to restrict the number of posters and decorative items depicting a dental motif, however, as this theme can easily be overdone. We are reminded of one young patient who entered the dental office, looked around in dismay, and remarked, "It's just too many teeth!"

Many dentists believe that children react negatively to white uniforms, but whether the dentist and his staff wear uniforms actually seems to make little difference to children. This was demonstrated in a study[9] in which 300 dentally inexperienced children, ages two to 15 years, were shown pictures of dentists in business attire, a white coat, and a conventional white clinic gown. When asked, "How would you like your dentist to look?", the children indicated no preference, thus dispelling the belief that children are negatively affected by the dentist's garb.

PREDICTING PROBLEM BEHAVIOR

One researcher who has studied children's dental behavior offered the following observation concerning children's responses to dental treatment.

> Essentially, a dentist has little to offer the young client except short-term pain and long-term gain. There is much about dentistry that is likely to maintain avoidance behavior by children in the dental setting. The dental operatory is unlike any of a child's natural settings —it is an environment in which the child lies on his or her back while two adults fill the mouth with numerous objects, some of

which make unusual noises, some of which cause unusual sensations, and some of which inflict pain. Lest any child remain calm, siblings and peers typically discuss and exaggerate many of their own adverse dental experiences just prior to a child's dental appointment. It is not surprising, therefore, that young children undergoing dental treatment frequently display a range of uncooperative behavior. . . .[10]

Weinstein[11] has calculated that child patients account for about 21 visits per week, or about one-third of the total number of patients seen in a week by the average dentist in general practice. When dentists are asked to evaluate the behavior of their child patients, they describe behavior problems with about six to seven percent of them. According to Weinstein, this means that the average general practitioner can expect to encounter management problems with one to two children per week, a fact which "signifies that a serious recurring problem exists for many practitioners."

Dentists themselves seem inclined to agree. A recent national survey[12] showed that many practicing dentists consider the uncooperative child patient to be among the most troublesome of problems in their clinical work. Uncooperative behavior interferes with the provision of dental care, increases the time necessary for delivery of care, and increases the risk of discomfort and injury to the child.

The Relationship Between Anxiety and Uncooperative Behavior

Among adult patients, uncooperative behavior during dental treatment is very rare because, as we noted in Chapter 4, even very fearful patients are mindful of social constraints on their behavior. Children, on the other hand, are more variable in their behavior. Young children, especially, are likely to "act out" their emotions, so a frightened child may cry, thrash about, try to escape, or even bite or kick the dental staff.

We noted earlier that most children express positive or neutral attitudes toward dentistry. However, about one-third of grade school children report some fear of dental treatment, and it is estimated that between six and 13 percent describe themselves as very fearful.[3,13]

Although fear and disruptive behavior often go hand in hand, this relationship is not perfect. Not all uncooperative behavior stems from fear and, conversely, not all fearful children are uncooperative. Every clinician has encountered children who, although obviously very tense, are nevertheless cooperative and compliant throughout the visit. Unfortunately, because their behavior does not hamper the dentist's ability to render care, these children can easily be overlooked. When working with such children, it is important to remember that they, too, need special attention, just as the child who expresses his fear in a more disruptive fashion. Special suggestions for working with these children are provided in the section on communicating with children. In addition, suggestions which apply to fearful children in general are appropriate for use with these children.

Variables Which Affect Fear and Behavior in the Dental Operatory

The identification of factors which contribute to children's fearful and disruptive behavior is worthwhile not only because this can help us predict which children might pose problems; more importantly, knowledge of these contributing variables may aid us in designing treatment methods to reduce problems of this nature. The factors which influence children's dental anxiety and behavior are varied. The important factors which have so far been identified are discussed in the following section.

Age, Sex, and Race   Among young children, the age of the child is one of the most important predictors of behavior in the operatory. In general, the younger the child the greater the likelihood of negative behavior. A mental age of about three years seems to be the dividing line between children who are able to accept dental treatment and those who are unable to do so.[14] Among children below three years of age, crying and negative behavior are to be expected. During the period from 34 to 48 months, fears increase and reach a peak.[15] Children in this age group often have trouble adapting to new situations, including the dental experience.[16,17] After 49 to 50 months of age, negative behavior diminishes and we can expect increasingly cooperative behavior.[17,18]

Among preschool and early elementary school children, there are no sex differences in cooperative behavior or fearfulness.[16,17] As children grow older, girls tend to describe themselves as more fearful than do boys, but there is no evidence that girls are less cooperative than boys.[13]

Cooperative behavior does not appear to be related to race; neither does the presence or absence of anxiety.[16]

Maternal Anxiety   In Chapter 4, we stated that an important source of dental fear is a negative family attitude toward dental treatment. Many clinicians have observed that children of very anxious mothers tend to be more fearful and less cooperative than children whose mothers do not describe themselves as anxious.

The research evidence strongly supports this observation. At the first dental visit, there is a very marked relationship between maternal anxiety about the visit and the child's anxiety and negative behavior during the visit.[19-22] Although this relationship has also been observed among groups of older elementary school children,[23] it appears to be most pronounced among children below the ages of 11 or 12 years. Some researchers have suggested that this relationship is present only at the initial visit, not at subsequent visits.[24,25] However, evidence on this point is inconclusive.

We should stress that this relationship is correlational and does not allow us to draw conclusions regarding cause and effect. While it may be the case that anxious mothers transmit their anxiety to their children, we can also argue the reverse. A mother who believes that her child is very apprehensive and likely to misbehave may respond to the dental visit with high levels of anxiety as a result of this knowledge.

Further, the relationship between maternal anxiety and child anxiety and behavior is not perfect. Not all anxious mothers have anxious children, and vice versa. Nevertheless, measures of maternal anxiety can be useful in helping to predict a child's response to the initial dental experience. These measures need not be elaborate: a simple question asking the mother to rate her own anxiety concerning the child's visit is sufficient. This information is likely to be especially useful when the child is young and/or dentally inexperienced and when the information is combined with other sources of information discussed in the following sections.

Socioeconomic Status   Study after study has shown marked differences between socioeconomic groups in their utilization of, and attitudes toward, dental treatment.[26-28] People of lower income and educational levels are less likely to obtain dental care on a regular basis. Instead, they tend to seek dental care when they are symptomatic. Dental visits, therefore, are likely to involve extensive and often painful treatment. One study,[26] for example, reported that, as income level decreases, the probability increases that the patient had extractions or oral surgery at his last dental visit.

With this in mind, we might assume that, as a group, people of lower socioeconomic status are more fearful of dental treatment than are people of higher income and educational levels. Many lines of research evidence support this assumption. Studies have shown, for example, that the lower the patient's socioeconomic status, the more likely he is to agree with statements relating to fear of the dentist.[6] Children from lower socioeconomic groups report significantly more dental anxiety[13] and tend to be somewhat less cooperative during treatment than children from upper socioeconomic levels.[21,29]

Past Medical Experiences   From knowledge of a child's past medical experiences, can we predict how he will behave at his first dental visit? If we know only the frequency of past medical visits or the length of time since the last visit, the answer to this question is, "No": this information alone is of little value in predicting behavior at the first dental visit.[21,22] If, however, we know whether past medical visits were painful or unpleasant, we are in a better position to predict the child's dental behavior.[21,22,30] As might be expected, children who have experienced painful or unpleasant visits to the pediatrician tend to be more fearful and less cooperative during the initial dental visit. The child's attitude toward medical people is also important: children who look forward to contacts with medical personnel without fear are generally more cooperative dental patients than children who anticipate medical visits with much fear.

Child's Awareness of Dental Problems   Several studies[21,22,30] have found a relationship between the child's belief that he has a dental problem and his behavior during the first dental visit. Children who believe they have a problem tend to be less cooperative during treatment than children who perceive no problems with their oral health. This tendency, which appears in both younger and older children, might reflect maternal anxiety transmitted to the child. Whatever the reason, these findings certainly lend support to the idea that children should have their first dental experience at an early age, before obvious dental problems develop.

Using Questionnaires to Predict Problem Behavior

Material in the preceding sections suggests that parents can provide much information that can be helpful in predicting the child's response to the initial dental visit. This information can be gathered easily by means of a written questionnaire, completed by the parent upon arrival for the initial visit. During the interview, this material can be reviewed with the parent. An example of a parent questionnaire is given in Figure 7-1.

Another important source of potentially useful information is the child himself. A variety of questionnaires have been used in the dental office to assess the child's feelings about the visit. A self-report measure that has proved quite useful was devised by Dr. Larry Venham.[31] Dr. Venham reasoned that young children do not have well-developed verbal or conceptual skills and that a questionnaire, even if read aloud to the child, might tax the abilities of the young patient. To avoid this, he devised a picture selection measure of anxiety for children. Pairs of cartoon figures, each differing in the type and intensity of the emotion portrayed, are presented to the child. The child is told to select the figure who feels most like the child himself feels at the moment. This test, which has been used with children ages two to 14, also has been shown to be valid and reliable. This task is suitable for routine office use and can provide valuable clues to a child's emotional state and the type of behavior that can be expected during treatment.

Please circle the answer which most closely applies

1. How do you think your child has reacted in the past to dental and medical procedures?*
   1. Very poor   3. Moderately good
   2. Moderately poor   4. Very good
2. How do you think your child will react to this procedure?*
   1. Very poor   3. Moderately good
   2. Moderately poor   4. Very good
3. How would you rate your own anxiety (fear, nervousness) at this moment?†
   1. High   3. Moderately low
   2. Moderately high   4. Low
4. Does your child think there is anything wrong with his (her) teeth such as a chipped tooth, decayed tooth, gumboil, etc.?†
   1. Yes   2. No
5. During the past year has your child been in contact with anyone who has had an unpleasant dental experience?**
   1. Yes   2. No
6. In the last two years my child's contacts with medical doctors have been . . .†
   1. Always enjoyable   3. Usually unpleasant
   2. Usually enjoyable   4. Always unpleasant
7. In the last two years my child usually looked forward to contacts with medical people . . .†
   1. With much fear   3. With no fear
   2. With little fear
8. In the last two years my child has experienced actual physical pain in connection with medical procedures.†
   1. Quite often (three or more times)   3. None
   2. Occasionally (once or twice)

FIG. 7-1. Maternal Questionnaire. * *Johnson, R. and Baldwin, D. C. "Relationship of maternal anxiety to the behavior of young children undergoing dental extraction."* J Dent Res *47(1968):801–5. Reprinted with permission.* † *Wright, G. Z. and Alpern, G. D. "Variables influencing children's cooperative behavior at the first dental visit."* J Dent Child *38(1971):124–8. Reprinted with permission.*

PREPARING PARENT AND CHILD
FOR THE INITIAL VISIT

As we have discussed, the initial dental experience can be a difficult and unpleasant time for some children. Hoping to minimize such problems at the first visit, clinicians and researchers have explored a variety of methods to prepare the child and his parent for the visit. Because these methods involve time, effort, and expense, it is important that we know which have been found to be most effective in bringing about reductions in anxiety and negative behavior.

The Preappointment Letter

How well do parents prepare their children for the first dental visit? This question is significant because, as we might expect, there appears to be a relationship between the child's dental behavior and the way in which his parents have discussed and explained the dental visit.[30] Children who are properly prepared tend to be more cooperative than children whose parents have failed to provide appropriate discussion and explanation.

Unfortunately, although research evidence is sketchy, available evidence suggests that parents may often do more harm than good in their attempts to help their child prepare for a first dental visit. In fact, one study showed that when parents attempted to alleviate child anxiety, many children actually became more apprehensive.[30] Obviously, a parent who does not know what the dentist really does or who believes that the dentist "pulls teeth" is not well equipped to prepare the child for the dental visit. Children prepared in this fashion tend to behave less cooperatively than children whose parents have explained that the dentist is someone who "fixes teeth" and prevents oral disease.

It is apparent that many parents could benefit from the dentist's assistance in the matter of preparing their children. Many dentists use preappointment letters for this purpose. Over 25 years ago, one clinician[32] reported beneficial effects of sending parents a preappointment letter and subsequent research has tended to support this method as helpful. When preappointment letters are sent prior to the first visit, mothers describe the letters as helpful,[33] child behavior tends to be more cooperative,[33] and there are fewer broken appointments.[34]

A preappointment letter need not be lengthy or complicated. It should welcome the parent and child and provide a brief explanation of what will take place at the first visit. It should also include suggestions for describing the dentist as someone who fixes teeth and helps them stay pretty and healthy. An excellent example of a preparatory letter, devised by Dr. Sylvan Mintz,[35] is shown in Figure 7-2.

One noted pedodontist[36] with many years experience working with children suggests that, in addition to a letter to the parents, the child himself be sent a card or note prior to the first visit. Children, he points out, typically receive little mail and are usually very pleased to receive mail addressed to them. This simple, inexpensive measure may help relieve a child's anticipatory anxiety and promote positive attitudes toward the dental visit.

Welcome,

I look forward to meeting you and your child at your first visit to my office. As a Pediatric dentist, my office and office routine may be somewhat different from what you have been accustomed to in the past. To have you and your child feel more at home, I would like to take a few minutes to familiarize you with my practice.

One of our prime objectives is to make your child a good dental patient who will be able to accept routine dental treatment. This process must begin at home prior to the first visit. Listed here are some suggestions to guide you:

1. Dental visits are part of growing up. Please don't offer rewards or indicate in any way that there is anything to fear.
2. The less "fuss" the better. It is best to tell a child about a dental visit the day of the appointment.
3. If your child requires more information, you can explain that the doctor will look at his teeth to make sure they are healthy.
4. Make appointment days easy and try to see that your youngster is well rested.
5. Don't threaten a visit to the dentist as punishment for misbehavior.

At the first visit, you will be asked to complete a medical and personal history questionnaire. Therefore, we would appreciate your arriving a few minutes earlier for this appointment.

The child at this visit is made acquainted with the dental office. He rides in the chair, sees how the water squirts, etc. He may have x-rays ("pictures") taken. If an irregularity in your child's bite is observed, impressions may be taken so that I can thoroughly study the condition. Everything that we intend to do is explained and shown to the child before we do it.

I encourage parents to accompany their children into the treatment area, especially children under five. The parent's presence is often comforting and reassuring in a new situation. Even on subsequent visits, the parent's presence is encouraged. It is important, however, for the parent to be a "silent partner," so that I can establish a good, direct relationship with the child.

If your child has a special toy, doll, or blanket that he or she would like to bring, please let him do so.

At the next appointment, your child's teeth are cleaned and a fluoride treatment is given. It is at this time, after the x-rays are interpreted and a complete examination has been completed, that your child's oral health, proposed treatment plan, and financial arrangements will be discussed. Please feel free to ask any question you may have.

My office is committed to a policy of prevention. By seeing your child early in life we can prevent dental decay and infections by early treatment, oral hygiene therapy, and diet counseling. Orthodontic problems can also be prevented or the severity lessened by early recognition and treatment.

Your child, with your cooperation, can become an excellent dental patient with a healthy mouth and a pretty smile.

Cordially yours,
Sylvan S. Mintz, D.D.S.

The Familiarization Visit

Some clinicians have advocated the use of a "get-acquainted" visit to the dental office prior to the initial exam or prophylaxis appointment. Such a visit, it is believed, helps to minimize the sense of strangeness and, hence, reduces the child's anxiety. Research evidence, however, has not strongly supported the effectiveness of a familiarization visit. In one study,[37] for example, maternal anxiety was reduced in the group that received a familiarization visit (probably due to the fact that mothers were explicitly told that the visit would help their children), but no effects on child behavior or anxiety were apparent. It is difficult, then, to argue that the additional expense and effort involved in a familiarization visit are really merited in terms of benefits gained.

Explanation and Exposure

While a special visit is probably not necessary, some preparation of the child before he enters the operatory for the first time does seem warranted. Clinicians and researchers alike have long focused on the use of explanation and exposure as a means of preparing children and introducing them to dentistry. The assumption that children, like adults, fear the unknown and gain comfort and security from knowing what to expect certainly makes sense. Further, this notion seems to be supported by findings concerning parental preparation of the child prior to the first visit.

The popular Tell-Show-Do method is a well-known example of an approach which employs information and explanation. Strictly speaking, it is not a preparatory method, as it is integrated through the entire sequence of procedures instead of being presented before the child actually enters the operatory. However, as it is chiefly an information/exposure method, we have included it in this section. The Tell-Show-Do method, as formalized by Addleston,[38] involves the following steps:

1. The dentist uses simple language to explain to the child what he is going to do prior to each procedure.
2. The dentist then demonstrates the procedure on himself or on an inanimate object.
3. When the dentist is sure the child understands what will be done, he begins the actual procedure on the child.

The Tell-Show-Do procedure is currently in wide use and, for this reason, it is especially curious that no research studies have been undertaken to

◀ **FIG. 7-2.** Letter to parents. *Mintz, S. S., in Levoy, R. P. "Success file: How to minimize those first-appointment anxieties." Dent Econ 68(1978):49. Reprinted with permission.*

evaluate its effectiveness. However, there are no indications that the method is in any way harmful or detrimental, so clinicians who employ this method can probably continue to do so without worry.

Recently, there have been attempts to use the Tell-Show-Do approach as a preparatory method, prior to entry into the operatory. The procedure has been refined so that anxiety-producing events are presented in graduated fashion. This format is similar to that used in systematic desensitization, but relaxation methods are not employed. Desensitizationlike methods have been used with both filmed and live demonstrations of procedures and techniques.

Research findings concerning desensitizationlike procedures with children are especially interesting because they illustrate the value of careful scientific evaluation of new behavioral methods and techniques. Logic, or "common sense," suggests that desensitization should be quite effective in reducing fearful, uncooperative behavior at the first visit. Yet results of several controlled investigations reveal that the method is not effective.[37,39-41] In fact, there are even indications that this approach can backfire. Dr. Barbara Melamed,[7] a noted authority on child dental behavior, found that a short demonstration film (four minutes) increased anxiety and uncooperative behavior in a group of four-to-11-year-old dentally inexperienced children. She concluded that approaches which focus on equipment and procedures can actually sensitize inexperienced children, making them more fearful and uncooperative than they might otherwise have been.

This finding may seem surprising, especially in light of the fact that adult patients respond well to desensitization and explanation. It is a rare occurrence, indeed, when desensitization results in additional sensitization in an adult patient. What has been overlooked, however, is the fact that children—especially young children—are limited in their verbal and conceptual abilities. An adult patient has not only a vocabulary which is many times greater than that of a young child; in addition, he has a lifetime of experiences which helps him to understand, imagine, and prepare for an impending new experience. The child's limitations in these areas suggests that we should expect only modest results, at best, from the use of explanation and information as a strategy for reducing children's fears.

Research studies of desensitizationlike methods are valuable for more than the negative findings concerning the effectiveness of these methods. When these studies are examined closely, an interesting pattern emerges. The results suggest that opportunities for friendly interaction with dental personnel outside of the operatory setting are more important than explanation or demonstration in preparing the child for dental procedures. In one study,[41] for example, one group of children spent several minutes in a conference room talking with a friendly dental assistant. Although this procedure was planned as a placebo control treatment, it actually produced considerable improvement in operatory entrance behavior when these children were compared with control group children and children who had been exposed to more formal preparatory methods.

Knowing the people, then, appears to be more helpful and comforting to a child than knowing the procedures. Fifteen minutes of the dental assistant's time spent chatting and getting acquainted with the child would seem to be time well spent. "Neutral territory," such as an office or conference room, should be used rather than the clinic operatory.

Modeling

Permitting children to watch other children calmly undergo dental treatment has long been advocated as a means of preparing the inexperienced child to accept treatment. This strategy not only teaches the inexperienced child what to expect; perhaps more importantly, it demonstrates what is expected of the child. Gerald Wright notes that it is surprising how many children do not really know what behavior is expected of them in the dental operatory. The dentist can, of course, explain the rules for office behavior but "A picture is worth a thousand words," and children are likely to derive much greater benefit from actually observing cooperative behavior than from merely hearing about it.

In fact, modeling has emerged as the most effective of the formal preparatory methods for eliciting calm, cooperative behavior in the dentally inexperienced child. Many dentists who work with children have reported the successful use of the patient's cooperative older brothers and sisters as models[35,42] and results of a controlled study[43] show that sibling models can indeed be helpful.

Of course, not all young children have older siblings available to serve as models. For these children, observation of other unrelated but cooperative children can serve as well, but care must be taken to ensure that only relaxed, well-behaved children are used as models. Since it is not always possible to arrange schedules so that such models are available, filmed modeling offers clear advantages.

As we noted in Chapter 4, filmed modeling is equally as effective as the use of live models. Several excellent studies of filmed modeling have shown that this method can produce considerable improvement in attitude and behavior of young, inexperienced dental patients.[23,44] With the availability of video equipment for home use, modeling films for children can easily be made in the dental office.

Preparatory Methods: Some Recommendations

From the preceding sections, we have seen that the likelihood of a successful initial visit is greatest when the child knows what to expect during the visit; knows and likes the dentist and his staff; and knows the rules for behavior in the dental office. Therefore, we recommend that a preparatory program for new child patients include all of the following:

- a previsit letter or booklet to help the parent prepare the child
- a get-acquainted period with the dental assistant in a nonclinic room
- a modeling film

For convenience, and because children become anxious if they are subjected to lengthy periods of waiting, the latter two ingredients might be combined. The dental assistant could watch the film with the child, then chat with the child and ask questions about the film.

IN-OPERATORY BEHAVIOR MANAGEMENT

Preparatory methods can be very helpful in minimizing management problems, but they do not always completely eliminate such problems. What additional measures can be employed in the operatory to further reduce the likelihood of problem behavior or to manage it if it should occur? Some specific questions which bear on this issue are: Is the parent's presence likely to be helpful or detrimental? Should rewards be given for cooperative behavior? What about criticism or the use of physical restraint if the child's behavior is disruptive? Can hypnosis be useful with child patients? We will discuss these questions and others in the following sections.

The Parent's Presence and Child Behavior

Every dentist who includes child patients in his practice must decide what his policy will be concerning the presence of the parent in the operatory. When given the option, most young children and their parents prefer to remain together, at least during the initial visits.[45] Yet the majority of dentists prefer to exclude the parent from the operatory and many feel so strongly about this that they would refuse to treat a child whose parents insisted on remaining with the child during dental treatment.[46,47] Dentists who prefer to exclude the parent believe that the parent's presence is disruptive and interferes with the dentist's attempts to develop rapport with the child, elicit cooperative behavior, and provide good quality dental care.

Dentists who prefer to have the parent remain in the operatory argue that parents can be a strong source of support and security for the young child. Notes one dentist[17] who has conducted research on this subject, "The child receives love and support from the mother from birth. To sever this relationship arbitrarily, at a time which represents a potential emotional and physical threat for children, seems unwise."

Certainly, clinicians can cite numerous examples supporting both sides of this argument. Venham describes mothers whose presence clearly provided strong support and security for the child. On the other hand, he also describes mothers who:

> . . . openly expressed fear of the dentist and specific dental proce-
> dures in front of their children and asked to avoid seeing the proce-
> dure. These mothers moved nervously in their chairs, hid their
> eyes, displayed exaggerated facial signs of fear, and emitted sounds
> associated with fear and anxiety, all in full view of their children.[48]

Research results have not supported the notion that the parent's presence increases patient management problems. In fact, although some studies
have reported no difference in child behavior with the parent present or ab-
sent, other studies have actually found significant increases in cooperative
child behavior when the parent was present.[17,48] Beneficial effects on child
behavior have also been obtained when an older sibling was permitted to
remain with the younger child.[44]

Research evidence, then, clearly indicates that it is to the advantage of
both dentist and patient to permit the parent to remain in the dental operatory during treatment. Of course, not all parents and children will wish to
remain together. Venham, for example, observed that remaining in the
operatory was stressful for some mothers who expressed feelings of frustration, helplessness, and fear that the child would feel "betrayed" by the
mother's inaction. This situation can be prevented if the parent is given an
opportunity to decide for herself whether she wishes to remain in the operatory.

If the parent chooses to stay, it is necessary to establish clear "ground
rules" to avoid potential problems. Parents sometimes assume that it is their
responsibility to deal with their child's fear or misbehavior in the operatory,
just as they would in other situations. This can be confusing to the child and
distracting to the dentist. For this reason, the parent should be told before-
hand that the dentist needs the child's undivided attention and that silent,
unobtrusive behavior on the parent's part will be most helpful to all concerned.

Hypnosis with Children

As anyone can testify who has ever watched young children make a
"house" from a blanket draped over two chairs or "travel to the moon" in a
discarded cardboard carton, children have vivid imaginations. The ease and
enthusiasm with which they enter into fantasy and "let's pretend" makes
them almost universally excellent hypnotic subjects.

In fact, on measures of hypnotic susceptibility, children obtain higher
scores than adults. Susceptibility seems to be at a peak between the ages of
eight and 12 years and begins to decline slightly thereafter.[49]

There are, of course, many differences between the child and the adult patient and these differences dictate some modifications in the hypnotic techniques employed. Because the child's attention span is shorter than that of an adult, children require more interesting and exciting induction procedures. Monotonous, repetitious procedures which are often useful with adults may lead to boredom and restlessness in the child.

Similarly, young children enjoy activity. They do not like to relax and suggestions for eye closure and relaxation usually meet with little success. Although children of seven to eight years of age can respond to suggestions for eye closure, it is not until about age 11 that they prefer to do so.[50] Extremely anxious children also prefer to keep their eyes open during hypnosis.

At what age can hypnosis be used with children? Some have suggested that hypnosis is not useful with children below the age of six. Others,[50] however, have demonstrated that children as young as three to four years old can respond to hypnotic inductions which consist of suggestions to fantasize involvement in a favorite activity.

Formal induction procedures are not always necessary with child patients, especially if the dental procedures to be performed are relatively minor, such as prophylaxis. Children respond very well to a technique known as "sensory confusion," a simple technique which consists of positively relabeling the sensations that the child will experience. Excellent results have been obtained with children undergoing prophylaxis merely by suggesting that the sensations caused by vibration of the hand-piece will be experienced as a tickling sensation.[29]

Distraction Techniques

The current trend toward quadrant dentistry has much to recommend it from the point of view of dentist and patient alike. Longer appointments allow the dentist to use his time in the most efficient fashion and mean fewer trips to the dentist for the child.

Although longer appointments do not seem to affect child behavior appreciably,[51] we must remember that children are action oriented and find it difficult to sit quietly for long periods of time. Even the most cooperative child patient can become bored and restless during a long appointment.

Videotaped material offers a very potent means of providing distraction during the time the child is in the chair. With the advent of reasonably priced video equipment designed for home use, a number of possibilities present themselves. A video monitor can be permanently suspended above the chair so that it is visible to the patient during treatment. Children become very excited at the prospect of seeing themselves "on television," and if a camera can be conveniently positioned, some children might be entertained for considerable periods simply by watching themselves on the monitor. Videotaped cartoons and other programs suitable for children can also be used. A library of tapes allows each child to select material of greatest interest to him.

The use of videotaped cartoons has been shown to produce significant improvement in the behavior of uncooperative children during dental treatment. Working with a group of very disruptive, uncooperative children, we[52] found that children whose rates of uncooperative behavior were in excess of 90 percent did not benefit from cartoon distraction.* However, for children whose rates of disruptive behavior fell between 50 and 90 percent (still very uncooperative and an unacceptable level for the provision of dental treatment), the use of videotaped cartoons resulted in significant reductions in uncooperative behavior.

If video recording equipment is not available, a regular television can be used, but this will limit the child's choice of program to what is broadcast at that particular time. Audiotaped songs and stories can also be used in place of television. The child can listen to taped material through headphones during treatment.

The Use of Reward and Punishment

In Chapter 6, we noted that consequences which follow a behavior play an important role in learning and we described the use of positive and negative consequences to produce changes in oral hygiene behavior. Can systematic use of immediate consequences also be helpful in teaching children to behave appropriately during dental treatment?

Unfortunately, we have only limited data on which to base a reply to this question because so little research has examined the use of this strategy in the dental setting. This is difficult to understand, as the use of contingent reward and punishment has proved extremely successful in changing a wide variety of other child behaviors and many have urged its use in the dental context.

In one of the very few studies[53] in this area, investigators worked with a group of severely retarded children whose behavior was so uncooperative that they had previously required restraints and general anesthesia. When fruit juice was used as a reward for sitting back in the chair and for mouth-open behavior, significant improvements in these behaviors resulted after two 45-minute training sessions. These results are very encouraging, but they do not constitute a true test of an in-operatory contingent reward program because the training program took place between dental visits rather than during actual treatment.

---

* Such children—rare among pedodontic patients above the age of four or five years—display out-of-control behavior that differs qualitatively from that displayed by less uncooperative youngsters. These children probably require additional management techniques, including between-visit training.

The use of aversive techniques in child management in the operatory is a controversial subject. Almost 90 percent of the postdoctoral pedodontic training programs in this country teach the use of techniques such as physical restraint and the so-called "hand-over-mouth" technique (use of a hand or towel over the mouth of a screaming child until the child quiets).[54] However, several writers have specifically cautioned against the use of aversive procedures, warning that the use of punishment is a risky undertaking. To understand why this might be so, we must examine the conditions under which punishment is most effective in producing long-term suppression of unwanted behavior.

A large body of evidence demonstrates that the effectiveness of punishment is directly related to its intensity. Mild punishment is usually ineffective in changing previously rewarded behavior; only when punishment is intense do stable changes in behavior take place. The ethical problems posed by this condition are obvious. Not so immediately obvious is the fact that intense punishment can lead to conditioned fear responses to any stimuli present at the time of the punishment—in our case, to all aspects of the dental environment, including the dentist himself. As Albert Bandura[55] states in a scholarly review of the topic, "The resulting avoidant responses may be more socially undesirable than the behavior the punishment was originally intended to reduce and, once established, they may be considerably more difficult to eliminate."*

Timing is also important in determining the effectiveness of punishment. Punishment is most effective if applied early in the chain of undesirable behavior. Since punishment, to be effective, must also be administered consistently, we face a dilemma. If punishment is reserved until the child engages in a full-blown tantrum, its effectiveness is reduced. The alternative, however, is to apply intense punishment for each instance of uncooperative behavior which might presage a tantrum. This alternative is quite obviously unacceptable.

Finally, research on the use of punishment procedures has shown that punishment can sometimes backfire and actually produce increases in undesirable behavior, especially tantrums and aggressive behavior. Recently, the same situation has been documented in the dental setting when criticism, blame, or coercive methods such as restraints have been used with disruptive children. In one study,[56] criticism for uncooperative behavior produced large increments in such behavior.† In contrast, an instructions-only proce-

---

* Recall that success rates for the treatment of dental fear remain lower than success rates obtained with other types of fear. Recall, too, that many fearful, avoidant dental patients give a history of rough or traumatic dental experiences.

† Recent research[57] suggests that the child's sex and previous dental experience may be important factors to consider. Inexperienced child patients and girls—experienced or inexperienced—respond especially poorly to criticism and verbal punishment.

dure, in which the dentist simply stated what the child should do, produced steady decreases in disruptive behavior. In another study[11] in which dentist–child interaction was the focus, dentist use of instruction and feedback was usually followed by compliant child behavior. On the other hand, attempts to control the child's behavior by physical or verbal force (threat, ridicule, blame, or physical restraint) were almost inevitably followed by resistant or uncooperative child behavior.

We have seen that serious problems accompany the use of aversive procedures. Because the conditions for effective punishment are so stringent, they are seldom met and punishment is, therefore, generally ineffective. Undesirable side effects and a "backfire" effect have been well documented and pose problems which cannot be lightly dismissed.

Why, then, do people continue to use punishment in an attempt to control behavior? Despite the long-term disadvantages, punishment often produces an immediate, if short-lived, change in behavior. This change is, itself, rewarding to the person who administers the punishment and makes it more likely that, confronted with undesirable behavior in the future, he will again use punishment to control the behavior.

Thus, the dentist who uses aversive methods to deal with tantrum behavior might obtain immediate results (the tantrum stops). He cannot, however, be certain that he is not producing undesirable side effects and even actually causing the behavior to increase in frequency over time.

COMMUNICATING WITH CHILDREN

In the course of our research and clinical work with children, we have often been struck by the changes which come over many adults when they interact with children. It is not unusual to observe people who are normally poised and socially skilled in interactions with other adults act in a forced and artificial fashion when talking with children. Some adopt a high-pitched voice, a sing-song cadence, or an effusive, "gushy" style. Others speak slowly and distinctly, as if the child were slightly deaf or not quite bright. Such changes in speaking style are neither necessary nor desirable. Your child patients will probably respond best if you address them in the same tone you use with your adult patients.

Of course, children do differ from adults in some important respects. Vocabulary and the ability to abstract are not well developed and the child's concept of time is limited. Young children, especially, live in the present and cannot project themselves into the future. Thus the statement, "If I fix your tooth now, it won't hurt you later," has little meaning to a young child.

Children are literal and concrete in their interpretations. They are sticklers for honesty and view a promise as sacred—as many a parent learns when it rains on the day of a promised outing and all attempts to reason with the child are drowned out by wails of "But you promised!" For this reason, be careful when you tell a child patient that you are "just going to look" at his teeth. Two experienced pedodontists, Drs. Till and Brearly,[57] point out that such a statement sharply limits your activities with the child patient. If the exam reveals the need for immediate treatment and you decide to proceed at once, the child will perceive you as untrustworthy and you will lose his confidence. To avoid this unfortunate situation, Till and Brearly suggest saying, "I am going to look at your teeth and then we will see if we have to do something more."

These authors also discuss the question of using a special vocabulary with child patients. Most schools teach dentists to substitute words such as "rubber raincoat" for rubber dam, and "sleepy water" for anesthesia. Till and Brearly argue that this terminology is nonprofessional and misleading. They urge that dentists, in their role as educators, teach children the meaning of words such as anesthesia, restoration, and preparation. There is no evidence available to support either side in this debate, so your own preference is the most useful guide in the matter. Of course, just as with adult patients, negatively charged words such as "pain," "hurt," and "needle" should be avoided and less threatening words substituted.

Whether or not you have used a modeling film to teach a child the rules of office behavior, direction and feedback should be provided throughout the session. Specific instructions concerning what the child is to do and immediate feedback have been shown to be more effective in avoiding problem behavior than coaxing, coercion, or rhetorical questions. Especially with young children, gentle physical guidance accompanying such verbal instructions as "hands in your lap" is often helpful in obtaining cooperative behavior.

The Shy Child

Adults often make the mistake of forcing themselves on shy children. Attempts to cajole or tease a shy child into responding are seldom successful and usually produce the reverse of the desired effect: the child simply burrows deeper into the safety of mommy's lap. In our own clinical work with children, we have found that such children "warm up" quickly if the professional initially focuses his attention on the parent. At intervals, without interrupting the conversation, a quick wink is directed at the child and attention is returned immediately to the parent. This initially produces retreat behavior in the child, who may turn away or hide his head. Few children resist for long, however. Soon the child watches intently for the next wink, then grins and giggles replace apprehensive looks. At this point, the clinician can begin to draw the child into the conversation.

Never try to tease or joke a child out of his anxiety. When you do, you communicate that it is—as he had thought—unacceptable to be afraid. The child will then double his efforts to hide his fear and, in the process, double his anxiety.

The Tense-Cooperative Child

The term "tense-cooperative"[58] refers to children who cooperate and follow all instructions but who show unmistakable signs of tension and apprehension. It is important to recognize the special needs of these children because tension renders them more sensitive to pain and discomfort. This, of course, increases their anxiety and a vicious cycle is established.

The tense-cooperative child needs to know that you recognize and accept his feelings and that you do not think less of him for feeling as he does. Because he is concerned about appearing "grown-up" and "brave," he will usually deny feeling afraid or scared (in his eyes, only babies are scared or afraid). However, observing aloud that he seems a little worried or tense ("grown-up" words) often makes it easier for the child to acknowledge his apprehension.

Do not, at this point, try to reassure the child by telling him, "It's all right to feel afraid," or "Lots of kids feel that way." In the first place, he probably wouldn't believe you. And, even if he believed you, his concern is his own fear, not that of "other kids."

Instead, tell the child that you can understand that he might feel nervous and that you know how unpleasant those feelings can be. Assure him that you will proceed very slowly and gently. You can safely tell him to raise his hand if he needs to stop and rest; these children virtually never abuse the hand signal.

SPECIAL PROBLEMS IN BEHAVIORAL PEDODONTICS

Of course, each of your child patients should be treated as a "special" patient and one who is important to you. Children, like the rest of us, tend to live up to expectations and greeting a child as "one of my best patients" or "one of my favorite patients" has been known to produce marked improvement in the behavior of not quite ideally behaved young patients.

Some children, however, present with behavior or needs which demand extra effort and care on the part of the dental team. These children, and some suggestions for working with them, are discussed in this section.

The Out-of-Control Child

The procedures described in the preceding sections are, in general, most effective when used as preventive measures. On the basis of available evidence, these methods appear to be useful for reducing the likelihood of fearful, uncooperative behavior in the inexperienced child and in managing milder forms of uncooperative behavior in all child patients, experienced as well as inexperienced.

For a small segment of the child patient population, however, these methods are not very effective. The behavior of these children, aptly described as "out of control," differs qualitatively as well as quantitatively from the behavior of mildly to moderately uncooperative children. Children who exhibit out-of-control behavior often begin to tantrum immediately upon entering the operatory or upon being seated in the dental chair. Their behavior quickly escalates in intensity as the dentist approaches to begin dental procedures. Such children do not merely cry or whimper; they scream and howl. They do not wiggle or fidget; they thrash, kick, and struggle valiantly to escape.

The out-of-control child can quickly tax the patience of the most even-tempered dentist and it is easy to become exasperated—even angry—after several minutes of trying unsuccessfully to quiet a screaming, thrashing child. Don't let yourself be lured into viewing the situation as a battle which you must win at any cost; the cost can be very high in terms of psychological trauma to the child and your own subsequent feelings of guilt and shame. We agree with Weinstein that it is probably better to end the session prematurely and/or to refer the child to another dentist than to risk the outcome of a pitched battle.

Sometimes, of course, it is not practical to refer the child to another practitioner, especially if your practice is located in a sparsely populated rural area with few dentists. What alternatives are available for the treatment of extremely uncooperative children?

Regretfully, we must acknowledge that the options are limited. At this time, we know of no behavioral methods which can be practically implemented during ongoing treatment procedures to produce rapid reductions in out-of-control behavior. Methods for reducing such behavior are available, as we have noted, but they involve the expenditure of additional time and effort. An effective program, for example, would probably require specially scheduled "training sessions" during which small groups of children observe live models, then receive rewards for gradually approximating the behaviors demonstrated by the models. It is obvious that little in the way of dental treatment could actually be accomplished during these training sessions and we do not believe that it is practical for a busy dentist to attempt to carry out a behavior change program himself. However, if the caseload warrants such an effort, a behaviorally trained psychologist might be retained as a consultant* to develop and implement behavior change pro-

---

* Community mental health centers, colleges, and universities usually have staff members qualified to serve in this capacity.

grams for very difficult children. Office personnel, after sufficient training, might eventually take charge of the program, conducting it themselves with occasional supervision from the consultant. Of course, you would charge a fee for this service, just as for any other service you provide to your patients.

The Resistant or Defiant Child

Some children openly communicate resistance or defiance with statements such as "No," or "I won't." Others use more passive but equally effective tactics such as averting their heads or clamping their jaws tightly together. While these children are more restrained in their behavior than the out-of-control child, they nevertheless challenge the dentist for control of the situation.

Some dentists attempt to deal with defiant behavior by coaxing and reasoning with the child. Others advocate meeting the challenge head-on with a firm approach, arguing that it is necessary to "call the child's bluff." Repeating instructions in a firm but neutral tone will sometimes bring results with defiant children, but advocates of the direct approach unfortunately do not describe what to do if the child is not, in fact, bluffing but is quite prepared to sit for hours with his jaws clenched and his head averted. In our experience, adult logic is seldom convincing to a six-year-old—except that, from the child's point of view, it is a useful maneuver to delay dental work. Physical struggles with the child are to be avoided at all costs; wrestling matches are undignified, unprofessional, and upsetting to all concerned.

If coaxing and coercion are ineffective (as they have indeed been shown to be), how can such children be managed? They can, of course, be placed in the same sort of "training group" used for out-of-control children, and, in fact, we would expect them to improve rapidly with such training. However, because this is an expensive approach, it should be reserved for those children who are very persistent in their defiant behavior.

A technique drawn from the work of family therapists can sometimes be useful for dealing with defiant children, especially in the hands of a dentist with a sense of humor. This technique involves the use of paradox, or, as a layman would describe it, "reverse psychology," because it involves instructing the child to defy you.

To use this approach, begin by reflecting the child's feelings with comments such as, "You don't like this one bit," and "You want me to know that you're really mad." When you have the child's attention, prescribe the behavior. Urge the child to continue to show you how angry he is; in fact, insist that he do so. Suggest modifications in his demonstrations: "Show me how mad you are. Stick your tongue out at me. That's right. Now, pound on the chair. Good!"

Most children, when confronted with these instructions, will initially respond by intensifying their defiant behavior. They quickly tire of this, however, because the behavior does not produce the desired effect of "stumping" the dentist. Some children will even see the humor of the situation and begin to giggle. Others will look puzzled or uncomfortable. In either case, insist that the child continue in his defiant behavior until it becomes obvious to you that he is willing to cooperate, even if his cooperation is a bit grudging.

REFERENCES

1. McElroy, C. M. "Dentistry for Children." *Calif Dent A Transact* 85, 1895. Quoted in Wright, G. Z. *Behavior Management in Dentistry for Children.* Philadelphia; W. B. Saunders, 1975.
2. Kleinknecht, R. A.; Klepac, R. K.; Alexander, L. D. "Origins and characteristics of fear of dentistry." *Am Dent A J* 86:842, 1973.
3. Morgan, P. H.; Wright, L. E.; Ingersoll, B. D.; Seime, R. J. "Children's perception of the dental experience." *J Dent Child* 47:243, 1980.
4. Barton, D. H. "The dental environment as seen by the child." *J Pedo* 1:26, 1977.
5. Rosenziveig, S.; Sforza, A.; Addelston, H. K. "Childrens' attitudes toward dentists and dentistry." *J Dent Child* 35:129, 1968.
6. Jenny, J.; Frazier, P. J.; Bagramian, R. A.; Proshek, J. M. "Parents' satisfaction and dissatisfaction with their childrens' dentist." *J Pub Health* 33:211, 1973.
7. Melamed, B. G. "Behavioral approaches to fear in dental settings." In *Progress in Behavior Modification,* Vol. 7. New York: Academic Press, 1979.
8. Swallow, J.; Jones, J.; Morgan, M. "The effect of environment on a child's reaction to dentistry." *J Dent Child* 42:43, 1975.
9. Cohen, S. D. "Children's attitudes toward dentists' attire. *J Dent Child* 40:285, 1973.
10. Stokes, T. F. and Kennedy, S. H. "Reducing child uncooperative behavior during dental treatment with modeling and reinforcement." *J Applied Behav Anal* 13:41, 1980.
11. Weinstein, P. "Identifying patterns of behavior during treatment of children." In *Clinical Research in Behavioral Dentistry: Proceedings of the Second National Conference on Behavioral Dentistry,* edited by B. D. Ingersoll and W. R. McCutcheon. Morgantown, W. Va.: West Virginia University, 1979.
12. Ingersoll, B. D.; Ingersoll, T. G.; McCutcheon, W. R.; Seime, R. J. "Behavioral dimensions of dental practice: A national survey." Unpublished manuscript, West Virginia University School of Dentistry, 1979.
13. Wright, F. A. C.; Lucas, J. O.; McMurray, N. E. "Dental anxiety in five-to-nine-year-old children." *J Pedo* 4:99, 1980.
14. Rua, B. *Proceedings of the 3rd International Symposium on Child Dental Health.* Copenhagen, 1971.
15. Gesell, A. *The First Five Years of Life.* New York: Harper and Brothers, 1940.
16. Shirley, M. "Children's adjustments to a strange situation." *J Abnormal Psychol* 37:201, 1942.

17. Frankel, S. N.; Shiere, F. R.; Fogels, H. R. "Should the parent remain with the child in the dental operatory?" *J Dent Child* 29:150, 1962.
18. Oppenheim, M. N. and Frankl, S. N. "A behavioral analysis of the preschool child when introduced to dentistry by the dentist or hygienist." *J Dent Child* 38:317, 1971.
19. Johnson, R. and Baldwin, D. C. "Relationship of maternal anxiety to the behavior of young children undergoing dental extraction." *J Dent Res* 47:801, 1968.
20. Johnson, R. and Baldwin, D. C. "Maternal anxiety and child behavior." *J. Dent Child* 36:87, 1969.
21. Wright, G. L. and Alpern, G. D. "Variables influencing children's cooperative behavior at the first dental visit." *J Dent Child* 38:124, 1971.
22. Wright, G. L.; Alpern, G. D.; Leake, J. L. "A cross-validation of variables affecting children's cooperative behavior." *Can Dent A J* 39:268, 1973.
23. Melamed, B. G. "Preparing children for dental treatment: Effects of film modeling." In *Behavioral Dentistry: Proceedings of the First National Conference,* edited by B. D. Ingersoll, R. J. Seime, W. R. McCutcheon. Morgantown, W. Va.: West Virginia University, 1977.
24. Klorman, R.; Ratner, J.; Arata, C. L.; King, J. B.; Sveen, O. B. "Predicting the child's uncooperativeness in dental treatment from maternal trait, state, and dental anxiety." *J Dent Child* 45:62, 1978.
25. Koenigsberg, S. R. and Johnson, R. "Child behavior during sequential dental visits." *Am Dent A J* 85:128, 1972.
26. American Dental Association, Bureau of Economic and Behavioral Research. *Dental habits and opinions of the public: Results of a 1978 survey.* Chicago, Ill., 1979.
27. Basic data relating to the National Institute of Health 1977. US Department of Health, Education and Welfare, Public Health Service, National Institutes of Health, DHEW Publication No. (NIH) 77–1261, 1977.
28. Infante, P. R. and Owen, G. M. "Dental caries and levels of treatment for school children by geographical region, socioeconomic status, race, and size of community." *J Pub Health Dent* 35:19, 1975.
29. Neiberger, E. J. "Child response to suggestion." *J Dent Child* 45:396, 1978.
30. Bailey, P. M.; Talbot, A.; Taylor, P. P. "A comparison of maternal anxiety levels with anxiety levels manifested in the child dental patient." *J Dent Child* 40:277, 1973.
31. Venham, L. L. and Gaulin-Kremer, E. "A self-report measure of situational anxiety for young children." *Ped Dent* 1:91, 1979.
32. Tuma, C. F. "How to help your child to be a good dental patient: An open letter to parents." *J Dent Child* 21:81, 1954.
33. Wright, G. L.; Alpern G. D.; Leake, J. L. "The modifiability of maternal anxiety as it relates to children's cooperative dental behavior." *J Dent Child* 40:265, 1973.
34. Hawley, B. P.; McCorkle, A. D.: Wittemann, J. K.; Van Ostenberg, P. "The first dental visit for children from low socioeconomic families." *J Dent Child* 41:376, 1974.
35. Mintz, S. S. Cited in Levoy, R. "How to minimize those first-appointment anxieties." *Dent Econ* 68:49, 1978.
36. Kielich, R. Personal communication, December 18, 1980.
37. Pinkham, J. R. and Fields, H. W. "The effects of preappointment procedures on maternal manifest anxiety." *J Dent Child* 43:180, 1976.

38. Addleston, H. K. "Child patient training." *Fort Rev Chicago Dent Soc* 38:7, 1959.
39. Herbertt, R. M. and Innes, J. M. "Familiarization and preparatory information in the reduction of anxiety in child dental patients." *J Dent Child* 46:319, 1979.
40. Johnson, R. and Machen, J. B. "Behavior modification techniques and maternal anxiety." *J Dent Child* 40:272, 1973.
41. Sawtell, R. O.; Simon, J. F.; Simeonsson, R. J. "The effects of five preparatory methods upon child behavior during the first dental visit." *J Dent Child* 41:367, 1974.
42. Gordon, D.; Terdal, R.; Sterling, E. "The use of modeling and desensitization in the treatment of a phobic child patient." *J Dent Child* 22:102, 1974.
43. Ghose, L.; Giddon, D.; Shiere, F.; Fogels, H. "Evaluation of sibling support." *J Dent Child* 36:35, 1969.
44. Melamed, B. G.; Weinstein, D.; Hawes, R.; Katin-Borland, M. "Reduction of fear-related dental management problems with use of filmed modeling." *Am Dent A J* 90:822, 1975.
45. Venham, L. L.; Bengston, D.; Cipes, M. "Parents' presence and the child's response to dental stress." *J Dent Child* 45:213, 1978.
46. Roder, R. E.; Lewis, L. M.; Law, D. B. "Physiological responses of dentists to the presence of a parent in the operatory." *J Dent Child* 28:263, 1961.
47. Ingersoll, B. D. and Tetkoski, M. "Dentist–patient communication: What do patients want to hear?" Unpublished manuscript, West Virginia University School of Dentistry, 1980.
48. Venham, L. L. "The effect of mother's presence on child's response to dental treatment." *J Dent Child* 46:219, 1979.
49. London, P. and Cooper, L. M. "Norms of hypnotic susceptibility in children." *Develop Psychol* 1:113, 1969.
50. Morgan, A. H. and Hilgard, J. R. "The Stanford Hypnotic Clinical Scale for Children." *Am J Clin Hypnosis* 21:148, 1978.
51. Lencher, V. "The effect of appointment length on the behavior of the pedodontic patient and his attitude toward dentistry." *J Dent Child* 33:61, 1966.
52. Zabin, M. and Ingersoll, B. "Use of video-taped cartoons with disruptive children in the operatory." Unpublished manuscript, West Virginia University School of Dentistry, 1980.
53. Kohlenberg, R.; Greenberg, D.; Reymore, L.; Hass, G. "Behavior modification and management of mentally retarded dental patients." *J Dent Child* 39:61, 1972.
54. Davis, M. J. and Rombom, H. M. "Survey of the utilization of and rationale for hand-over-mouth (HOM) and restraint in postdoctoral pedodontic education." *Ped Dent* 1:87, 1979.
55. Bandura, A. *Principles of Behavior Modification*. New York: Holt, Rinehart and Winston, Inc., 1969.
56. Melamed, B. G.; Bennett, C.; Hill, C. J.; Ronk, S. "Strategies for patient management in pediatric dentistry." In *Clinical Research in Behavioral Dentistry: Proceedings of the Second National Conference on Behavioral Dentistry,* edited by B. D. Ingersoll and W. R. McCutcheon. Morgantown, W. Va.: West Virginia University, 1979.
57. Melamed, B. G. "Operant procedures in the management of children's disruptive dental behaviors." In B. Ingersoll (Chair): *Behavioral Approaches to Dental*

Fear, Pain, and Stress. Symposium presented at the meeting of the Society of Behavioral Medicine, New York, 1980.
58. Till, M. J. and Brearley, L. J. "Communicating with children." *NW Dent* 49:392, 1971.
59. Lampshire, E. L. *Control of Pain and Discomfort: Current Therapy in Dentistry,* Vol. 4. St. Louis: C. V. Mosby, 1970.

8

Special Problems of the Geriatric Patient

ASUMAN KIYAK AND JAMES BENNETT

WHY SPECIAL CONSIDERATION OF THE ELDERLY?

A major criterion of successful aging is how well the individual maintains oral aesthetics and oral health, the ability to chew, the ability to talk, and personal satisfaction with oral health status. Unfortunately however, the mouth often becomes one of the first areas of the body to be neglected among people who suffer chronic disease and infirmities in old age. It thus becomes part of the downward cycle of neglect, depression, and further neglect. As a dentist, then, you are therefore often faced with dental problems that may be closely related to the patient's other diseases and/or emotional problems.

To the 23 million elderly persons in America who have spent an aggregate of approximately two billion dollars to maintain their mouths and receive dental care over a lifetime, one of the greatest ironies is the increased risk of oral disease when the individual can least afford treatment and is often unable to maintain his personal oral hygiene. The increased incidence of oral disease, complicated by other factors such as physical and socioemotional disorders and increased problems in maintaining personal hygiene, suggest that dentists must focus on the special needs of older patients.

As the dental I.Q. of the population increases, we will find more and more people maintaining some or most of their natural dentition throughout the life cycle. The dental team is already faced with a new segment of the population for treatment planning and staging dental care. Future generations of elderly will have more knowledge about dental care and greater expectations of the dental team. They will present mixed dentitions which require more thoughtful treatment planning and staging than does the edentulous or fully dentulous mouth. No longer will geriatric dentistry be equated solely with prosthodontics. Specialists in oral medicine, periodontics, and endodontics, as well as general practitioners have already begun to face the unique problems of aged patients. The primary goal of this chapter is to provide a wider perspective on some of the special aspects of geriatric dentistry.

Another reason for greater emphasis on geriatric dentistry is the changing age structure of the U.S. population. The number of persons aged 65 and older has increased dramatically in the United States. With a declining birthrate, the elderly represent the fastest growing segment of the population. In addition, we are becoming an older society as the median age continues to increase.

The purchasing power of elderly persons will probably not change appreciably into the next century as inflation undermines fixed and inadequate retirement pensions and social security benefits. Older people will find their buying power significantly decreased; greater pressure will be placed on government agencies to include dentistry in Medicare and other national health insurance plans. At the same time, economic adversity will restrict the extent of health care provided by federal and state governments. As the cost of health care continues its steep rise, it is highly probable that dental auxiliaries will play a greater role in treating the elderly. Denturists may also be expected to provide low-cost prosthodontic services for some older patients. At the same time, however, a well-trained general practitioner or specialist will still be required to provide most dental services to the elderly. Health care providers in hospitals, nursing homes, and other institutions have already recognized the importance of dental care for the elderly as part of the patient's total care. Hence, there will be greater demands on the dental team to provide services in institutional settings.

Having presented some demographic and health care projections which are expected to influence future geriatric dental care, let us now focus on specific characteristics of the elderly. The social, cognitive, and perceptual status of aged persons and their typical medical and psychological conditions will influence their oral health. Finally, the dental care provider and the patient's environment (living arrangement, financial status, other health care providers) impinge on the quality of oral health services and health maintenance for the elderly. Figure 8-1 illustrates this dynamic model.

Before proceeding with this chapter, a word of caution is offered. Although we will describe characteristics of the elderly in general terms, it is impossible to characterize the "typical" aged person. More than any other age group, the elderly represent tremendous diversity in their physiological, social, psychological, and economic status. While some elderly fulfill the stereotype of the ill, confused, and isolated aged, many others are active, healthy, and independent. Within this range lies a diversity of older persons.

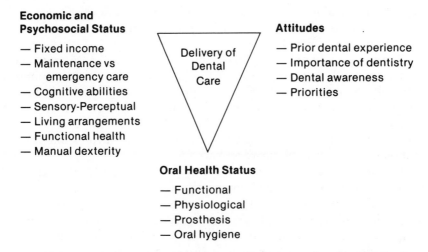

Economic and Psychosocial Status

— Fixed income
— Maintenance vs emergency care
— Cognitive abilities
— Sensory-Perceptual
— Living arrangements
— Functional health
— Manual dexterity

Delivery of Dental Care

Attitudes

— Prior dental experience
— Importance of dentistry
— Dental awareness
— Priorities

Oral Health Status

— Functional
— Physiological
— Prosthesis
— Oral hygiene

FIG. 8-1. Variables which influence dental care for the elderly.

Even with this caveat, however, two basic assumptions may be made about the elderly. These assumptions form the framework for the material in this chapter. More specifically:

- Aging represents survival. Those who live to be 75 have survived the diseases of youth and middle age which killed their less hearty peers. These survivors may live to a very old age with multiple "battle scars" (i.e., chronic diseases) which may eventually limit their daily activities. Nevertheless, the mouths of the elderly reflect the many years of stressful onslaught of microbes, nutrients of questionable value, iatrogenic dentistry, and the like.
- As we grow older, our lifespace becomes more constricted because of social changes (e.g., retirement, widowhood) and physiological changes (e.g., decline in physical endurance and sensory-motor skills). Likewise, the mouth becomes less able to tolerate these increased stressors.

Social Status of the Elderly
The population over 65 is now 23 million, or 11 percent of the total U.S. population.* Demographic projections suggest that this growth rate will accelerate well into the 21st century.

When one considers the differential lifespan of men and women 69 and 75 years, respectively, it is not surprising that the majority of persons over age 65 today are female. At age 65, there are 79.4 men for every 100 women in the United States. This proportion drops to 62/100 by age 75 and 48.5/100

---

* All population figures and percentages in the text are taken from the most recently available U.S. Census figures (1975, 1980).

at age 85. The majority of women over age 65 are widowed and live alone. They continue to live independently in the community and report frequent contact with children and friends.

The majority of older men live with a spouse in the community. They are predominantly retired, although surveys indicate 30 percent continue to work full- or part-time. Retirement represents a major role change for many elderly and often leads to reduced income and changes in lifestyle. Although several researchers have explored the impact of retirement on health, there is little evidence that retirement produces depression or other psychological or physical disorders.[1]

Despite stereotypes, only a small proportion of elderly are institutionalized. Indeed, those in nursing homes represent just 4.5 percent of all aged persons. The great majority of home care is provided to elderly by relatives.[2] Although older people are not very likely to become institutionalized, the number of disabilities and chronic conditions increases with age. The majority have at least one chronic disease. Nevertheless, more than half of the elderly report their activity level to be quite high. Only 16.4 percent indicate they are unable to carry on major activities.[3] The tendency to reduce activities because of chronic conditions is greatest in nonwhite elderly, those with less than five years of education and $3,000 annual income. Clearly, these are the individuals who have received the least preventive health care in their youth and are the most disabled in their later years.

The median income of families headed by older persons is lower than that of any other age group. In 1975, this was $8,057, while that for older persons living alone was $3,655. This is somewhat above the poverty level, although disproportionate numbers of elderly women and blacks have incomes below poverty. Indeed, 96 percent of older black women in families had incomes that classify them as poor.

It has been estimated that, in order to maintain their lifestyle after retirement, older couples with no children at home must have retirement income equivalent to 75 percent of their preretirement income.[4] Among today's elderly population, fewer than one-third have any income besides Social Security, which replaces only 45 percent of preretirement income for couples and 30 percent for individuals. Thus, nearly all aged persons experience a decline in real income after retirement. It is therefore not suprising that many elderly seek part- or full-time work. Approximately 18 percent work full-time, but in so doing, they lose a significant portion of their Social Security benefits. Federal legislation is pending which will reduce (but not entirely stop) penalizing elderly who work by limiting their Social Security eligibility. With the growth of private pension plans, it is possible that in the future the elderly will not experience the severe loss of income which restricts one's lifespace and one's social and psychological well-being, a condition which is all too prevalent in today's population of elderly. One of the major implications of limited income in the later years is reduced health care. Services which are not covered by Medicare (particularly dental and preventive health care) are often ignored.

Psychological Status of the Elderly

The study of the psychology of aging encompasses several areas: sensory-perceptual and psychomotor processes, cognition, drives, motives, personality, and social processes. While each of these topics deserves detailed discussion, it seems most critical for the dental team to be aware of changes in sensory-preceptual, motor, and cognitive functioning with aging. For this reason, we will discuss these changes in this section. In the bibliography at the end of this chapter you will find sources which offer more detail on the psychological status of the elderly.

Sensory–Perceptual Changes   Probably in no other area of psychology is the clinical and research evidence so conclusive: As we get older, we simply cannot see, hear, touch, taste, or smell as well as we did when we were young. We should note at the outset that decline in all five sensory channels begins relatively early. We reach our optimum capacities in our twenties, maintain this peak for a few years, and gradually decline. The rate of decline varies across the five senses and across individuals. Visual acuity, for example, seems to decline rapidly after age 45, while our olfactory capabilities are often maintained into the seventies. Because these changes are gradual, we adapt and use compensatory mechanisms as each sensory mode weakens. We rely on other, still–intact systems, stand closer to people and objects we want to hear or see, utilize nonverbal cues such as touch and different body orientations, succumb to bifocals and hearing aids. However, internal and external compensatory mechanisms become more difficult if the decline in any one system becomes severe or if all the sensory channels deteriorate concurrently.

Most age-related changes in vision are attributable to changes in the cornea, lens, and retina. Accommodation, or the ability to focus from near to far, declines with age. The lens grows denser and loses elasticity. The lens may become totally opaque and permit no light to enter. The incidence of cataracts increases with age, although even among 80-year-olds, the incidence is quite low. Despite the debilitating impact of cataracts, a solution is readily available today. Surgical removal of the damaged lens is a common procedure with a high success rate, even for the very old. Other visual problems associated with aging are decreased sensitivity to some colors, greater susceptibility to glare, problems with low light levels and dark adaptation, as well as reduced depth perception. Increasing sensitivity to glare is attributable to increased opacity of the lens with age, to change in curvature of the cornea and irritation of the cornea, and in some cases to increased turbidity of the vitreous.

Turning now to hearing, it is recognized that the most common cause of auditory deficiency in old age is "presbycusis," or progressive bilateral loss of the ability to hear high frequency tones. It is estimated that 16 percent of the 65-and-over population in the United States suffers from advanced presbycusis,[5] although more than half have mild loss of hearing. Individuals who have been exposed to high volume and high frequency noise throughout their lives (e.g., urban dwellers, factory workers) show more decline in old age than those from rural, low-noise environments. It is for this reason that women generally show less decline than men. To some extent, one may compensate for a loss in hearing high frequency tones by increasing the volume. This is the principle behind the hearing aid design. One of the difficulties with this approach, however, is the concomitant increase in volume of background noises. Another compensatory mechanism is to isolate the stimulus from background noises, or at least to eliminate as much of this background as possible. This is particularly important when we realize that the inability to hear high frequency tones greatly reduces one's speech discrimination ability.

Research in taste and smell modalities is somewhat more equivocal than in hearing and vision. While most researchers agree that taste sensitivity begins to decline after age 55, differences in their research methods may have produced different results. Richter and Campbell[6] found older adults between ages 52 and 82 needed higher concentrations of sucrose to identify its sweet taste than did children and younger adults. Similar results have been found[7,8] with the other three primary taste qualities, although sensitivity to sour and bitter tastes declines later. More recent researchers have used psychophysical procedures and found only minimal change,[9] although Hughes[10] did find a steady decrease in taste sensitivity. Medications, especially in high doses, may also alter taste sensations and the ability to enjoy food.

Evidence for decline in olfaction is even more contradictory. Even some studies reporting age-related loss found significant individual differences.[11] Some researchers have suggested that age per se may change olfactory and taste sensitivity, but health and smoking may affect outcomes.[12] Reduced taste and olfactory sensitivity may significantly lessen the ability to enjoy food. This problem is aggravated if the older person also experiences declines in visual and auditory functions. These factors contribute to reduced appetite and interest in food, thereby resulting in poor nutrition and poor dietary habits in old age.

Psychomotor Functioning   Although the incidence of mobility problems is greater among the elderly, age per se does not cause motor disabilities. Disease states such as arthritis, stroke, some cardiac disorders, and damage to the kinesthetic sense may affect both the peripheral and central mechanisms responsible for mobility. It has been estimated that one in every five persons over 65 has some limitation in the activities of daily living, although only five percent are confined to bed. The remaining 15 percent can get around with mechanical assistive devices or by relying on others' help.

Maximum strength and stamina for continuous exertion declines among many elderly. Maximum strength at age 70 has been found to be 64.4 percent to 83.6 percent of the maximum capacity of a 25-year-old. This drops to 50 percent by age 80, although elderly who maintain an active physical fitness program show much less decine in strength. Other factors limiting mobility include stiffness of joints, reduced ability to turn the neck, difficulty in gait and posture. Finally older persons have generally been found to have slower reaction times, both in simple and choice reactions tasks. While several hypotheses have been offered to explain this decline, including decreased speed of nerve impulse conduction, neuronal loss, and decreased blood flow, current data are inconclusive in providing answers to this important area of age-related decline.

Cognition Popular belief supports the position that aging does not affect immediate memory and memory for the distant past. Laboratory studies have supported the former hypothesis and showed that little if any age-related decline occurs in immediate memory. It is considerably more difficult to study memory for the distant past. It may be that rehearsal of significant events aids in their storage. In contrast, short-term memory in the elderly is affected when information is presented rapidly, exposed briefly, and frequently interrupted.[13] When material is presented in a structured manner, elderly are no worse on retention and recall of new information than are young persons.

Although the elderly have been found to experience problems in verbal learning, this may be related to differences in memory and reaction time and to reduced risk taking rather than a normal decline in learning ability. Elderly in good health and high I.Q. levels have been found to maintain this ability. Problem-solving behavior also shows some deterioration in the elderly. The reasons for this should be readily apparent from our earlier discussions: slower reaction time, susceptibility to interference and stimulus overload, deficits in short-term memory, rigidity and reduced abstract thinking skills.

In summary, it appears that some changes in sensory-perceptual, psychomotor, and cognitive processes are due to normal aging. Many other changes, however, are attributable to secondary processes such as disease and environmental conditions, and to increased caution of the aged person in responding to a stimulus. Accommodation, acuity, depth and color perception are the major visual changes with aging. Reduced ability to hear higher frequencies and need for greater concentrations of odors and tastes also occur in the later years. Physical strength declines and reaction time increases, while short-term memory, verbal learning and problem solving show some age-related decrements.

Physiological and Medical Status of the Elderly

Only recently has research on physiological aspects of aging gone beyond comparisons of young college students and institutionalized elderly. These studies found, not surprisingly, consistent differences between young and old, with the latter possessing only a fraction of the functional capacities of the former. Since 1955, a series of longitudinal studies have been conducted at the Gerontology Research Center,[14,15] at the National Institute on Aging,[16,17] and Duke University's Center for the Study of Aging.[18,19] These projects have examined longitudinally persons between 20 and 96 for periods ranging from five to 20 years. These data sets provide group means on normal, age-related changes in physiological functioning.

The primary findings of these studies are:

1. Physiological changes after age 65 are gradual
2. There is a steady decline with time, but older persons can function well even with 50 percent of their organ system and tissue capacity
3. Not all persons age at the same rate physiologically
4. Within each individual, different systems age at different rates.

An important change is a decreased ability to respond to stress and to return to homeostasis. It appears that even those elderly whose resting heart rate and blood pressure are similar to the young have more difficulty returning to normal levels after stress than would a young person. That is, reserve capacity declines in old age, thereby increasing recovery time following stress. This is also true in temperature regulation, which results in greater likelihood of hyperthermia and hypothermia for the aged.[20]

There is a steady decline after the mid-twenties and thirties in the efficiency of all physiological mechanisms, with rapid decline after the mid-sixties.[14] Perhaps the most notable is a decline in breathing efficiency because of declines in maximum breathing capacity, residual lung volume, and basal oxygen consumption. This affects metabolic rate, which declines by 20 percent between age 30 and 90 because there is less oxygen to combine with nutrients to produce energy, amino acids and glucose. This results in decreased reserves for other physiological functions.

Cardiovascular functioning declines in most persons with age. The heart pumps harder but achieves less, resulting in less cardiac output. The arterial wall rigidifies, myocardial contraction lessens, and peripheral resistance declines. These structural changes may produce inaccurate measurement of blood pressure with traditional methods. Research suggests that systolic blood pressure increases after age 65, but diastolic pressure does not.[21] Shock[22,23] notes that blood plasma flow may be expected to decrease by 55 percent between ages 30 and 80. In addition, renal blood flow, glomerular filtration, and tubular excretion rates decrease.

There is some conflict regarding the extent of decline in digestion and absorption in the gastrointestinal tract with age. However, it seems clear that hydrochloric acid and other digestive fluids decrease with age; ptyalin is reduced by 20 percent, trypsin by 30 percent, and pepsin by 20 percent. Motility in the intestine and colon declines, contributing to the problem of constipation in old age. Another area of change is hormonal activity. Decreases in hormones which promote immunity may affect the synthesis of antibodies and may be a major factor in age-related chronic diseases.

Bone physiology also changes with old age because absorption rate exceeds deposition, resulting in a net loss of bone. There is a progressive thinning of bone walls and decreased overall skeletal mass. This produces the common problem of frail and brittle bones in old age; osteoporosis represents a severe loss of bone mass. The process appears to be compounded in postmenopausal women and Caucasians. It appears related to calcium becoming less available for deposition because of factors which inhibit calcium absorption and metabolism, or an imbalance in the calcium/phosphorus ratio. The practical outcomes of these skeletal changes is increased risk of fractures and crushed vertebrae, resulting in a shortened, outward-bowing spine, as well as a shortened rib cage which may restrict respiratory functioning. Decreased calcium metabolism and absorption may also affect the older person's dentition and supporting alveolar bone.

There is unequivocal evidence that morbidity, particularly chronic diseases, increases with age. Normal age-related changes such as increased blood pressure and decreased glucose tolerance may result in pathological conditions for some elderly but not all. In contrast, minor dysfunctions of middle age may produce serious disease in old age. This includes obesity and anemia, which may compound other conditions in old age such as hypertension, diabetes mellitus, and respiratory diseases. Coronary heart disease also increases in the later years; with a doubled mortality risk for males after age 45 and tripled risk for females. Thus, while cardiovascular disease accounts for 39 percent of deaths between age 45 and 64, it accounts for 50 percent after age 65. This includes cerebrovascular accidents, the incidence of which increases markedly with old age. Of the 200,000 deaths from strokes each year in the United States, 80 percent occur in the elderly.

Among pulmonary diseases, chronic bronchitis, fibrosis, and emphysema increase significantly with age, four times as often in men as in women. Allergic responses increase, especially to drugs and bacterial products. This may be compounded by the use and misuse of multiple drugs among the elderly. Asthmatic conditions persist in old age and may contribute to pulmonary emphysema and respiratory insufficiency.

The incidence of arthritis and osteoporosis also increases with age. The former affects 14 percent of all males and 23 percent of females beyond age 45, limiting the victims' activity. Osteoporosis is four times as common in women and is a painful, debilitating condition which is only now becoming better understood. Osteoarthritis represents the third most common disorder of middle age, following obesity and hypertension.[24]

Impact on the Dental Care Provider

The description provided above of the social, psychological, physiological, and medical changes observed in many elderly has several implications for dental care providers. First, it is clear that the aged represent a diverse population group, with varying socioeconomic and psychological characteristics. Nevertheless, they are generally likely to be poorer, have less expendable income for health care (especially dental care), less likely to be working, and more likely to be widowed. While their functional health is often good enough for them to maintain an independent lifestyle, it is important that we recognize some characteristics which limit their access to dental care. Their living arrangement, limited income and social supports, and unavailability of transportation, make it more difficult for the aged to obtain dental services.

Sensory-perceptual changes, primarily in visual and auditory modalities, demand sensitivity from you and your staff in communicating home care instructions, description of services, and costs. Decrease in psychomotor ability will also reduce the aged person's level of oral hygiene maintenance. Specifics of communication with aged patients are provided in the following section. Changes in other sensory modalities, as well as some medical conditions, means a change in nutritional patterns. Poor dietary habits, often compounded by social isolation, are a factor in poor oral health and hygiene. Nutritional foods may not taste as strong to the aged palate, may require more time and energy to prepare, and their cost may seem too high for elderly on a fixed income. Insufficient knowledge regarding nutritional requirements often combines with these problems, resulting in inadequate intake of calcium, iron, and protein.[25-27] It is, therefore, critical that you conduct periodic dietary assessments of your older patients. If poor nutrition appears to be affecting the patient's oral health, the social, economic, and perceptual reasons must be determined.

The role of pathological aging on oral health is one of your principle concerns. Of special importance is an understanding of the impact of cardiovascular, circulatory, or arthritic conditions upon oral health maintenance and disease, as well as on patient management. A thorough medical evaluation and consultation with the aged patient's physician is imperative—considerably more so than for younger patients. This must include a comprehensive survey of all the medications a patient is presently taking, both prescribed and over-the-counter, those taken several times a day as well as those the patient takes only occasionally. Because of the greater likelihood of allergic reactions in old age, you must evaluate the patient's potential reaction to any medications you prescribe. Remember, too, to consider the interaction of these drugs with the patient's other medications.

Finally, you will need to determine whether the aged patient's chronic diseases and medications may influence treatment in your office. That is, does the patient have physical access to the office? Is he or she ambulatory or does he or she require mechanical or physical assistance? Can he or she tolerate long appointments? What about positioning the patient in the dental chair? This is particularly problematic for patients with neurological or muscular disorders.

In this section, we have presented a framework for considering the special needs and characteristics of the elderly. Through a better understanding of these issues, the dental team can better provide oral health services to an increasing population of elderly and can become leaders in comprehensive, appropriate health care for this segment of our population. We now turn to a discussion of some important dental problems of the aged and the role of health care providers in resolving these diseases.

KEY ISSUES IN THE DENTAL MANAGEMENT OF OLDER PATIENTS

When we consider the dental management of older patients, several issues emerge. We must, of course, be knowledgeable concerning the most common and the most important types of dental problems among older people. We must also be aware of important issues in interactions between the dental team and the older patient and between the dental team and the community.

Dental Problems of Older Patients

Dental Plaque Diseases   Dental decay and periodontal disease are the most pervasive, silent, and deleterious entities affecting a patient's remaining natural dentition. Dental caries commonly initiates on the root surfaces; if it remains hidden in an interdental area, the entire crown may suddenly disappear. With current interest in maintaining some healthy root structure in alveolar bone, it may become necessary to develop a DMFR (decayed, missing, filled, root) index for epidemiological studies of the elderly. The dental stereotype of the nursing home patient is one who enters the institution with a reasonable combination of natural teeth and prostheses; within one to two years, the natural teeth become decayed root tips and affect the fit of prostheses. Any time an elderly patient has significant decay on an abutment tooth maintaining a bridge or partial denture, the situation should be considered urgent; consider the cost of altering or making a new denture, bridge, or partial.

For the older patient whose periodontium has survived the onslaughts of middle age, the aging process may chronically destroy one or two teeth at a time. The economics of periodontal therapy versus prosthetics becomes a very cogent factor when we consider the fact that up to 80 percent of elderly patients with remaining teeth may have periodontal disease.[28] All of the complexities of aging must be considered:

1. Altered stress reactions
2. Insufficient or inappropriate nutrition
3. Altered immunocompetency
4. Altered ability to control plaque.

Periodontitis is probably the most common dental disease entity that forces the dentist to plan and stage the patient's treatment very thoughtfully.

Another important dental plaque problem is the seeding of oral bacteria into the blood stream. This can be life threatening in patients with rheumatic heart disease, prosthetic heart valves, artificial joints, dialysis patients, and the like. Problems like these will continue to grow in the elderly population as medicine continues to advance.

Chewing Dysfunctions   The ill-fitting denture is the classic dental problem of the elderly. It is a problem in which the nutritional, emotional, and social consequences may be devastating. Although remaking dentures is a popular solution, very viable alternatives lie in relines, soft lines, or even permitting the mouth to remain edentulous.

Soft Tissue Problems   Squamous cell carcinoma is obviously the most significant oral soft tissue problem for the elderly. Fortunately, it is much less common than many benign soft tissue lesions. Although its overall incidence is estimated at four percent, it occurs most commonly in the sixth and seventh decades.[29] Unfortunately, oral cancer is usually very painless in the early stages, and in its developmental stages it cannot be distinguished from other benign processes. It is the dentist's affective style with older patients that is so extremely important in managing any oral lesions; cancerophobia may easily be induced or exacerbated.

Other common soft tissue problems are cheek biting; varicosities of tongue, lips, and cheeks; redundant tissues beneath dentures; ulcerations; keratosis; and general atrophy of the mucosa.

Iatrogenic Problems This section refers not only to dental-related problems, but also to a wide range of physiological and/or emotional reactions that any health care provider may have precipitated. Some iatrogenic problems arise from inattentiveness to such things as medical workups or poor intraoral exams, while other problems arise from poor restorative care.

In dentistry, examples of the less serious iatrogenic problems arise from restorative procedures that may create future problems (e.g., overhangs or poor contacts). In prosthodontics, placing the patient in an excess retrognathic jaw relation may create TMJ pain where none had existed before. More serious problems arise from neglecting to assess the medical status of the patient before major drugs are prescribed. A current example of "double indemnity" lies with heart valve patients whose heart must be protected by antibiotics. Blood clotting ability must be assessed before invasive dental procedures are begun.

Planning and Staging Dental Care
Perhaps the key issue in geriatric dentistry is listening to the patient, hearing what he says as well as what he hesitates to say, and the way he expresses it.

The dentist–patient relationship is one of the most important elements for achieving acceptable maintenance of oral health. The ability of the dentist to provide reasonable quality of care and the ability of the patient to comply with treatment planning, preventive oral health measures, and dental care follow-through, are behavioral interactions that are often complex since relatives, friends, clergy, physicians, lawyers, estate trustees, and others frequently become involved at various levels of decision making.

The elderly represent perhaps the most heterogeneous age group of all. Their attitudes, levels of trust, and acceptance range from "You're the boss, Doc," to "Just pull out this one," to a suspicious, "You're a dentist, huh? What are you here for? To pick up my spare change?" With the more dependent elderly, arriving at a dental care plan will require more time for explanations, questions to understand the patient's needs, and consultation with family members.

The burden of responsibility falls heaviest on the general dentist who, as the primary dental care provider, must orchestrate and coordinate the patient's dental care; he/she is often faced with developing alternative care plans when the patient's social, financial, or health status is compromised.

From the dentist's side of decision making, it is often a problem of staging the care to fit the patient's medical, emotional, and economic status. From the patient's viewpoint, it is often an extremely variable range of expectations that may have very little balance with reality, deeply influenced by childhood and young adulthood experiences with dentistry. The 80-year-old, white-haired great-grandmother may still experience the same conditioned autonomic reactions she had as a teen-ager in the dental chair, particularly if she had some harrowing experiences in a dental office 60 or 70 years ago.

Economics is also a key issue; it has an impact on treatment planning and staging. Among the major problems are the following:

- Elderly are not covered for dental costs by Medicare; those who have Medicaid often find it to be inadequate.
- Many elderly are not aware that they qualify for Medicaid or are reluctant "to go on welfare." As a result, 96 percent of dental costs for the elderly are paid by private funds.[30]
- Only 1.6 percent of the aged person's income is devoted to dental care.[12] This is a reflection of the low utilization rate for the elderly; 50 percent have not seen a dentist in five years. Elderly report seeking dental care "only when needed."[30]

The dentist is usually deeply imbued with the concept of ideal treatment planning, often because the educational and training environment seldom gives him/her adequate breadth and depth in staging dental care (e.g., providing care in a time frame and environment that best fits the patient's medical, emotional, social, and economic situation [in addition to his/her dental complexities]). Probably most dentists can recall those treatments that would have been entirely different had one or more of the above-mentioned factors been given greater consideration.

Primary dental care may be defined as:

1. Those measures which intercept, slow down, or halt the process of dental pain, infection, or dysfunction;
2. Those procedures which provide basic function and esthetics appropriate to the patient;
3. The involvement of the patient in a home maintenance and recall program (i.e., continuity of care).

It is important to recognize that primary care for some elderly patients will require extensive restorative procedures, while for others complete extraction with no prostheses may be the best. The decision to perform conservative versus extensive dentistry will demand sensitivity: What is the patient's physical health status? What is his cognitive and emotional status? Does he have any motor disabilities which will limit personal maintenance of oral health? Can this aged patient come to the dental office on his own, or can he rely on friends and relatives for transportation? Can you provide mobile dental services if the patient needs it, or refer the patient to another practitioner with such services? With such extreme heterogeneity in all characteristics of the elderly, the dental team should be flexible and oriented toward serving the patient's needs.

Planning and staging care for the elderly will become a more critical issue for the dental team as more elderly relocate from independent living situations to institutional care (e.g., hospitals, rehabilitation centers, long-term care facilities). It is often the dental assistant and/or hygienist who can best provide the dentist with perspectives that strengthen the planning and staging process, especially in institutional settings. Thus, we must ask: What role should the dental auxiliary play in providing oral health maintenance to the elderly? Can the background and training of all dental personnel be expanded in this area? That is, can the functions and responsibilities of auxiliaries be expanded in geriatric dentistry while the dentist better prepares himself to make decisions regarding dental treatment in the face of significant medical, emotional, and social factors? The future dental care of the elderly will be dependent upon efficient, humanistic, and cost controlled dental care by a team.

It is the aim of this chapter to help you become more aware of the diverse social, psychological, and physiological factors which make the elderly patient different from young and middle-aged patients. Their often complex and compromised oral health status provides a challenge to the most experienced dentist. Yet, the dramatic changes which can be produced in the aged patient's oral, physical, and psychological well-being with even minor restorative treatment suggests that such a challenge is well worth taking.

REFERENCES

1. Atchley, R. C. *The Social Forces in Late Life.* Belmont, Ca.: Wadsworth, 1976.
2. Wilder, M. H. "Home care for persons 55 years and over: United States, 1966 to 1968." *Vital and Health Stat* Series 10 No. 73, 1972.
3. Wilder, C. S. "Limitation of activity due to chronic conditions: United States, 1969 to 1970." *Vital and Health Stat* Series 10 No. 80, 1973.
4. Henle, P. "Recent trends in retirement benefits related to earnings." *Monthly Labor Rev* 95:12, 1972.
5. Corso, J. F. "Auditory perception and communication." In *Handbook of the Psychology of Aging,* edited by J. E. Birren and K. W. Schaie. New York: Van Nostrand Reinholt, 1977, pp. 497–534.
6. Richter, C. P. and Campbell, K. H. "Sucrose taste thresholds of rats and humans." *Am J Physio* 128:291, 1940.
7. Byrd, E. and Gertman, S. "Taste sensitivity in aging persons." *Geriatrics* 14:381, 1959.
8. Cooper, R. M.; Bilash, I.; Zubek, J. P. "The effect of age on taste sensitivity." *J Geront* 14:56, 1959.

9. Hermel, J.; Schönwetter, S.; Samueloff, S. "Taste sensation identification and age in man." *J Oral Med* 25:39, 1970.
10. Hughes, G. "Changes in taste sensitivity with advancing age." *Geront Clin* 11:224, 1969.
11. Kimbrell, G. and Furchgott, E. "Effect of aging on olfactory threshold." *J Geront* 18:364, 1963.
12. Chalke, H. D.; Dewhurst, J. R.; Ward, C. W. "Loss of sense of smell in old people." *Pub Health* 72(6):223, 1958.
13. Botwinick, J. *Aging and Behavior.* New York: Springer Publishing Co., 1973.
14. Shock, N. W. "The physiology of aging." *Scient Amer* 206:100, 1962.
15. Shock, N. W. and Andres, R. "Adaptive responses to glucose in elderly males." In *Adaptive Capacities of an Aging Organism,* edited by D. F. Chebotarev. Kiev, USSR: Academy of Sciences Publications, 1968.
16. Birren, J. E. *The Psychology of Aging.* Englewood Cliffs, N.J.: Prentice-Hall, 1964.
17. Birren, J. E.; Butler, R. N.; Greenhouse, S. W.; Sokoloff, L.; Yarrow, M. R. *Human Aging: A Biological and Behavioral Study.* Washington, D.C.: Government Printing Office, 1971.
18. Palmore, E. *Normal Aging: Report from the Duke Longitudinal Study, 1955–1969.* Durham, N.C.: Duke University Press, 1970.
19. Palmore, E. *Normal Aging II: Report from the Duke Longitudinal Study, 1970-1973.* Durham, N.C.: Duke University Press, 1974.
20. Pickering, G. W. "The peripheral resistance in persistent arterial hypertension." *Clin Sci* 2:209–35, 1936.
21. Masero, E. J. "Physiologic changes with aging." In *Nutrition and Aging,* edited by M. Winick. New York: John Wiley & Sons, 1975.
22. Shock, N. W. "Physiologic aspects of aging." *Am Diet A J* 56:491, 1970.
23. Shock, N. W. "Physiological theories of aging." In *Symposium on the Theoretical Aspects of Aging,* edited by M. Rockstein, M. L. Sussman, J. Chesky. New York: Academic Press, 1974.
24. Sharp, C. and Keen, H. *Presymptomatic Detection and Early Diagnosis.* London: Pitman Medical Publications, Ltd., 1968.
25. DHEW. *Ten-State Nutrition Survey, 1968-1970.* DHEW Pub. #HSM72-8133, Center for Disease Control, Atlanta, 1972.
26. DHEW. *Preliminary Findings of the First Health and Nutrition Survey, 1971–1972.* DHEW Pub. #HRA74-1219-1, Washington, D.C., 1974.
27. Steinkamp, R. C.; Cohen, N. L.; Walsh, H. E. "Re-survey of an aging population." *Am Diet A J* 46:103, 1965.
28. Schaefer, W. G. and Waldron, C. A. "A clinical and histopathologic study of oral leukoplakia." *Surg Gynecol Obstet* 112:411, 1961.
29. Tiecke, R. W. and Bernier, J. L. "Statistical and morphological analysis of 401 cases of intraoral squamous cell carcinoma." *Am Dent A J* 49:694, 1954.
30. Gift, H. C. "The seventh age of man: Oral health and the elderly." *Am Coll Dent J* 46(4):204, 1979.

9

Considerations in Care of the Patient with a Disability

DORIS J. STIEFEL AND D. ELOISE STULL

If you practice in an average community in the United States, you and the other dentists in your community will be treating an increasing number of disabled persons. It is estimated that there are presently between 33 and 36 million persons in the United States, that is, 15-16 percent of the population, who experience a serious limitation in activity. This means that one out of six patients in your patient pool may have a major physical or mental problem. While the type or severity of the disabilities will vary, all will have affected the life of your patient as far as mobility, activity level, ability to work, self-image, and attitude toward health care are concerned.[1]

In recent years, significant increases have occurred in the size of our population of disabled citizens. The advances of medical technology have not only resulted in a higher initial survival rate for people born with disabilities or who acquire them during their lives, but have also lengthened their life expectancy. Moreover, the life span of the population as a whole has lengthened, and as persons age, their medical problems increase proportionately.

Persons with disabilities are also becoming more mobile, both physically and socially. As part of an ongoing process of normalization, they are becoming increasingly integrated into the general community. A concerted effort has been made of late to bring the disabled out of isolation, away from institutions and into the mainstream of society. Halfway facilities, group homes, and independent living centers are offering the support services needed to assist deinstitutionalization and encourage independent living. In recognition of the universal right of disabled persons to an active and rewarding life, 1981 has been declared the "International Year of Disabled Persons."

The societal changes in attitude toward disability will inevitably be reflected in your dental practice. Historically, "special patients," that is, those persons who for reason of their physical or mental difficulty require special consideration, have all too often not received adequate dental care. The dental profession is now recognizing that it must take an active role in correcting past neglect and meet its responsibilities towards the underserved segments of our population. It is, indeed, significant that the American Dental Association adopted as its theme for 1980, "Access—Dentistry's Answer."

As you begin to treat patients who are disabled, you will realize that the disease process and dental procedures for these patients are essentially the same as for all patients. What then makes treatment of the disabled patient unique? It is the fact that in caring for such patients, the dentist and the dental auxiliary will not only need to perform the technical tasks of restoring the oral cavity to optimum health but must come to know and understand the patient as an individual, whose lifestyle is circumscribed by his/her disability. Much more than with the average able-bodied patient, successful management of the patient with a disability requires the dental professional to have a sound knowledge of the psychosocial and medical issues affecting that patient.

For example, whereas the healthy person is expected to take responsibility for seeking dental care, keeping appointments, making payments, and complying with instructions on oral hygiene, some disabled patients may be incapable of carrying out such normal obligations of a dental patient. Depending on the functioning level, he/she may be totally dependent on others to perform them. As a consequence, the dentist will need to relate appropriately not only to the patient but to the patient's family and all those involved in the patient's care. Counseling the patient, guiding him/her to essential services, and coordinating dental procedures with other therapies may all be part of the dental problem plan.

Dentistry for the special patient is a challenging and rewarding experience. It is well to remember that the vast majority of disabled patients can be treated in the regular private dental office setting. By becoming familiar with the characteristics of the major disabilities and the associated psychosocial issues, and by learning to treat patients thus affected, you will build up the necessary confidence and lay the foundation for a practice open to all types of patients, disabled as well as able-bodied.

WHO ARE THE DISABLED?

What kind of an image does the term "handicapped" or "disabled" call to mind for you—a child with Down Syndrome, a resident of an institution, someone who moves awkwardly or is in a wheelchair, or an individual on a street corner with a Seeing Eye dog?

Certainly, persons with a disability encompass all of the above. It must be realized, however, that included also are individuals of all ages, from all walks of life, and of every level of intellectual functioning. Their impairment may be readily visible to the observer, it may be less apparent as in the case of deafness, or it may be a hidden problem such as a serious systemic disorder.

One of the reasons for the apparent disagreement in demographic data is the difficulty in determining objective criteria for what constitutes a handicap or disability. Many persons, in spite of serious problems, do not wish to consider themselves in such terms. Perhaps the best guidelines are those specified in federal legislation. As stated in the Rehabilitation Act of 1973, a "handicapped person" means any person who:

- Has a physical or mental impairment which substantially limits one or more major life activites, such as caring for one's self, performing manual tasks, walking, seeing, hearing, speaking, breathing, learning, and working.
- Has a record of such an impairment (has a history of, or has been misclassified as having a condition that limits major life activities).
- Is regarded as having such an impairment.[2]

A corollary of the above definition is that limitations in major life activities must be considered in terms of age and occupation of the individual. Thus, for the child with cerebral palsy, the inability to participate in the normal play or school activities of his/her peers would constitute a substanial handicap. The middle aged homemaker with multiple sclerosis, who finds herself unable to perform formerly routine tasks of meal preparation and housekeeping, certainly faces a major disability. Similarly, the 75-year-old who, as a result of a stroke, can no longer perform personal hygiene tasks, including tooth brushing, is also severely handicapped.

The extent of a person's handicap is dependent on the degree to which his ability to function normally has been affected. Indeed, this concept is fundamental to an understanding of the disabled person's attitude towards his problems. It explains why the term "disability" is preferred rather than "handicap." While the latter is widely used in official terminology, it has certain negative connotations. Persons with a disability think of themselves as impaired in a specific area of functioning, such as mobility or loss of one of the senses, but fully able to function in other areas of daily living.[3] They feel that the emphasis should be on their abilities rather than their disabilities and on themselves as individuals. The old medical joke about "the gallbladder in Room 304" is insensitive; unfortunately, however, this approach to a label rather than a person is often a reality.

At the same time, disabled persons recognize that they have certain problems in common and constitute a minority who, like other minorities, are demanding their rightful place in society. One major difference distinguishes this population from other disadvantaged groups; it is a minority of which anyone can become a member. It is sobering to ponder the fact that most of us who presently belong to the "normal" majority are in reality only temporarily able-bodied; if we live long enough the chances are considerable that we, ourselves, or a member of our immediate family will suffer a permanent major disability.

For years there have been organizations for specific disabled populations (i.e., blind, deaf, multiple sclerosis, muscular dystrophy, cerebral palsy). These organizations have offered support and information to the disabled population and their families. Recently, significant change has taken place; these specific groups have joined in coalition to present uniform needs of persons with disability. As a result, the rights of disabled persons to the same opportunities as able-bodied people have been officially recognized in the United States and are guaranteed by Section 504 of the Rehabilitation Act of 1973. The regulations to this act ensure that no otherwise qualified person shall, by reason of his handicap, be discriminated against in the areas of education, employment, or social services, including health care.[4]

For the dental practitioner Section 504 has obvious implications. The regulations require that a dentist who accepts any federal payments, such as Medicaid, cannot withhold services from a patient solely to make reasonable person's disability. If, after full evaluation and an effort to make reasonable accommodations, the dentist feels unqualified to treat a particular disabled patient or the dental office is physically not accessible, the dentist has the obligation to refer that patient to another practitioner who is able to provide the necessary care. As an illustration, consider the following scenario. Dr. Jones enters his operatory, prepared to treat his next patient, Susie, a little girl seated quietly in the dental chair. One glance tells him she has Down's Syndrome. He mumbles something, walks out without any attempt to examine her, and two minutes later his assistant informs Susie's mother, "I'm sorry but Dr. Jones does not treat retarded children." This situation is no longer permissible. If Dr. Jones normally includes children in his practice, he should have made an effort to treat Susie. If her dental or general management posed problems beyond his capabilities, he should at that point have referred her to another more qualified dentist.

For dental clinics receiving federal monies and employing 15 or more people, the law is more stringent. In addition to the general obligation of nondiscrimination, the program of care must be physically accessible to the wheelchair-bound and appropriate auxiliary aides must be provided (i.e., interpreters for deaf patients).

BARRIERS TO DENTAL CARE

Adequate dental care has been termed the greatest unmet health need of the disabled.[5] Multiple factors are known to play a role in the poor oral health status of many persons with handicaps.

Yet, for the most part, it is not the disease process per se which is different in these persons*; rather the difference lies in the amount of care received. A review of studies comparing dental disease in developmentally disabled children and young adults with nondisabled control groups revealed no significant differences in caries prevalence. However, the amount of restorative care was less, oral hygiene tended to be worse and, concomitantly, periodontal disease more severe in the disabled groups.[6,7] Clearly, the major problem is one of dental neglect.

While it has been emphasized that the disabled do not constitute a homogeneous population, it is useful in our evaluation of the dental patient with a disability to note some characteristic problems. Thus, people with severe handicaps frequently are psychosocially disadvantaged. In addition to the specific physical or mental impairment, they tend to experience difficulties which act as deterrents to dental care.

Such barriers fall into a number of categories:

- Difficulty in physical access
- Financial constraints
- Poor motivation
- Lack of qualified and willing dental professionals to provide care

The physical problems in accessing dental care are multiple and profound. In 1977, approximately 6,770,000 persons were reported as limited in mobility. The rate of mobility limitation increases with age; not surprisingly, it is inversely related to income.[8] Disabled persons frequently are dependent on others for transportation. If a cabulance or ambulance is re-

---

Certain exceptions should be noted; e.g., an increased susceptibility to severe periodontal disease is associated with Down's Syndrome. Individuals with Down's Syndrome and cerebral palsy also tend to have a higher prevalence of malocclusion. Gingival hyperplasia is a common side effect of dilantin therapy for seizure disorders.

quired to bring the patient to the dental office, considerable expense is incurred over and above the cost of the treatment itself.

Many dental offices are not designed for persons who have severe ambulation problems or are in wheelchairs. The patient who has recently lost the use of his legs through trauma or disease may suddenly discover that the familiar dental office, which he has visited for many years, has become completely inaccessible to him because it is on the upper level of a building without an elevator.

The effect on dental care of such limitations is borne out in a survey of homebound patients. In this study, 78 percent of the 269 patients responding to a questionnaire on their perceived dental needs reported it was difficult or almost impossible to get to the dentist. A strong positive correlation was shown between the ability of homebound patients to go the dentist and the time elapsed since the last dental visit.[9]

Financial Constraints

Dental care may be financially extremely burdensome, if not beyond reach, for many disabled persons. According to the Bureau of the Census, income and activity limitations are inversely related. In 1971, the median income of disabled persons was 60 percent that of the nondisabled,[8] and for the severely disabled, it was 40 percent.

Statistics for subgroups of the disabled population tell an even more compelling story. Persons 18 to 64 years old who are work disabled tend to have less formal education than those without limitations. The unemployment rate is also twice as high for the disabled group as for the able-bodied. The problems are worse for blacks than for whites, with over 70 percent of severely disabled blacks as compared to 40.6 percent of whites living near or below the poverty level. Whereas less than one-fifth of nondisabled persons live on public income maintenance, almost one-half of the generally disabled and almost two-thirds of the severely disabled are supported by such funds.[8]

Compounding the problem are the higher health related expenditures for disabled persons. As a group, in 1972 they spent 2.5 times as much for medical care and 3.5 times as much for hospital care as the nondisabled population.[8] A severely disabled individual may also have ongoing medical supply needs. As an example, an individual with a spinal cord injury will need wheelchair repair and replacement, daily supplies to manage bladder and bowel, plus medications.

In contrast, dentistry is usually considered an elective health care service. Unlike hospital and physician services, most dental fees must be paid from private funds and—as might be expected—utilization of dental services is directly related to income. Coverage for dental care under Medicaid (public assistance) varies from state to state and, at the present time, Medicare (Social Security) has no provision for routine dental treatment. Moreover, a considerable number of disabled persons "fall between the cracks"; they may earn a very low income, in a sheltered workshop, for example, which will disqualify them for public assistance, yet they will not be able to afford dental services.

Inadequate Dental Motivation
In view of the severe problems in mobility, economic deprivation, and lower educational levels of many disabled persons, it is no wonder that dentistry is often accorded a low priority in the health needs of handicapped persons. There are usually too many more immediate problems.

Consider, for example the family who struggles to make both ends meet, where there are several children at home demanding attention, and Mother has to take Johnny, who is multihandicapped and a management problem, several times a week for medical therapy. She is unlikely to seek dental treatment for Johnny unless it is made logistically and financially simple for her, preferably as part of the overall care plan. Nor is she likely to have much energy left for brushing Johnny's teeth or, indeed, be too interested in their condition; after all, she herself expects to wear dentures in a few years. Besides, it is easier to keep Johnny quiet and content if she gives him his favorite candy bar.

Lack of dental awareness or concern extends beyond the disabled individual and the immediate family to other members of the community, both professional and paraprofessional, involved in his care. The director of the long-term care facility, for example, may not be dentally oriented and the facility may have staff and funding problems. Usually assistance with personal hygiene is the duty of the aides, who tend to be poorly educated, possibly suffer from dental neglect themselves and are often reluctant to brush their charges' teeth.

As dental professionals, you have a vital and leading role to play in educating and enlightening all those concerned with the disabled person's health. It is up to you to motivate attendants and responsible persons to practice good hygiene habits and to seek professional dental help for the individuals in their care. While the principles of disease prevention, early intervention, and the importance of good oral health apply universally, there are important differences which must be stressed concerning the individual with a disability.

- The disabled person, by reason of physical or mental impairment, often is dependent on others for the performance of daily hygiene tasks including brushing and flossing of the teeth.
- If dental health is permitted to deteriorate, the consequences may be far more serious and costly for the disabled than for the able-bodied patient.

Supposedly Johnny, our multihandicapped youngster, is now 25 years old. His dental history has been one of emergency care only. He is brought to the dental clinic from his group home 30 miles away by cabulance, an expensive mode of transportation. He permits only a cursory examination which reveals decay, missing teeth, extensive plaque, and periodontal disease. His health history includes a congenital heart defect, which puts him at high risk for endocarditis from dental infection. Since Johnny is unlikely to tolerate dentures, and because of his systemic condition, it becomes important to arrest the disease process and retain as much of his dentition as possible. He will require prophylactic antibiotic coverage before any dental procedures are done. In view of his behavioral problems, the extensive nature of the treatment required, and the difficulty in transportation, it is decided to schedule Johnny for general anesthesia. How much better if the added health risk and cost factors involved for this patient could have been avoided through early interception of the disease process through regular dental care, a behavior management approach, and better attention to plaque control.

Dental prevention for the disabled patient is clearly an area in which the joint efforts of the full dental team (dentist, dental hygienist, and dental assistant) will be most effective. It also provides an exciting opportunity for the dental team to work in concert with the larger body of interdisciplinary care providers concerned with the patient's well-being. In this way, dentistry can make a significant contribution to the disabled individual's health, well-being, and ability to function.

Lack of Qualified Dental Professionals

The founding in 1948 of the Dental Guidance Council for Cerebral Palsy marked the advent of organized professional endeavors to meet the dental needs of the disabled. Prior to that time, persons with handicapping conditions generally had such a short life expectancy that dental care was not a relevant issue.[10] The poor prognosis applied not only to congenitally afflicted individuals but also to those impaired through trauma. Accustomed as we have become to seeing quadriplegics and paraplegics increasingly participate in the everyday life of our society, we are shocked by the fact that not one person with spinal cord injury survived from World War I to World War II.

For the most part, dentistry for the disabled patient was considered the realm of the specialist, particularly the pedodontist, who had had advanced training in this area, and of the few general practitioners who had developed an interest in this field and had gained their experience without the benefit of formal education. It was only in the 1970's that demonstration projects supported by the Robert Wood Johnson Foundation at eleven American dental schools showed that undergraduate dental and dental auxiliary students could, indeed, satisfactorily learn to treat special patients. Since that time, other dental schools have begun to incorporate courses in care of the disabled patient into their teaching programs and curriculum guidelines have become established.[11]

The opportunities for undergraduate students to gain knowledge and skill in this area of dentistry has important long-range implications for the availability of dental care for the disabled population. A number of studies have shown that dentists who received clinical or classroom instruction or had previous experience in care of handicapped patients tended to include them in their practices.[12,13] Conversely, those who did not treat them most often cited lack of competence as the reason. Dental students who had participated in a special course on disabilities scored consistently higher on confidence tests after the course than before the course. Their predominant attitude was a practical one and remained unchanged: "Will work with those patients with whom I feel capable."[14]

Confidence in the ability to treat a patient appears to be the determinant of whether that person will receive care. The more knowledge and clinical experience in treating various types of disabled persons you acquire as a student, therefore, the more confident you will become in meeting the challenges of the special needs patient and the more likely you are to include such a patient routinely in your future practice.

ATTITUDES TOWARD DISABILITY

Considerable attention has been given to the attitudes of nondisabled persons toward physically disabled persons. Gellman's theory states that society's approach to the disabled individual involves a variety of historical attitudes: the ancient Greek belief that disabled people were inferior; the preprophetic Hebraic idea that the sick were being punished by God; the early Christian faith that the disabled person had acquired moral virtue.[15]

Each of these historic beliefs can be seen in today's attitudes toward persons with disabilities. The person with the disability is often regarded as inferior, not only with respect to specific ability, but as a whole person. Frequently, persons with disability find themselves spoken for, as if they were not present or were unable to speak for themselves. As an example: a man in a wheelchair due to spinal cord injury told of an experience in a restaurant where his wife was asked, "And what does he want for dinner?" People with disabilities are also often treated as children. A quick review of film titles about persons with disabilities ("Joey," "Larry," "Joni," and "Charlie") communicates the message that disabled individuals are young. Many times, professional individuals who are disabled are inappropriately addressed by their first names rather than by their professional titles.

The preprophetic Hebraic belief that the sick are being punished by God is an attitude that is very subtle. However, many adult-onset disabled individuals "buy into" this belief. "Why me?" "What have I done to deserve this?" are unanswerable questions. Other inquiries of "What happened to you?" or "How did you get that way?" connote a sense of responsibility. The actual question may not imply personal responsibility; however, at times the tone of the question makes one feel the need to explain that it was not a personal responsibility. Taking responsibility for an illness is a common response. Zola reported on a college class assignment in which students were asked to describe (as if to a five-year-old) their last illness. Each student accepted responsibility for his own illness. For example, a student reporting about a cold stated, "I went out in the rain without a coat and then I caught a cold." Illness was paired with a mistake or error.[16]

Conversely, the suffering-saint syndrome or "I don't know how you do it" attitude prevails. Persons with disability may be identified, correctly or incorrectly, as having many positive personality traits. Using experimental methods, Mitchell and Allen had the same individuals role playing in two counseling sessions; first, as a nondisabled counselor and second, as a counselor in a wheelchair. They reported the disabled counselor received a more positive rating on empathetic understanding, level of regard, and congruency.[17]

People with disabilities have experienced a wide variety of attitudes. A common experience is to encounter a range of subtle and not-so-subtle prejudices. Sayer surveyed 682 sophomore students from Northeastern University on social attitudes of university students toward the disabled. The conclusions of this study suggest that students who had previous contact, i.e., friends or family members who were disabled, tend to have more favorable attitudes and that the degree of tolerance is related to the extent of contact. Females tend to demonstrate a more positive attitude than males, and individuals who pursue a major field of study that is people and/or service oriented seem to develop more positive tolerances.[18]

As health care providers, the questions that face all of us are: "What is my attitude toward persons with disabilities; do I have prejudicial attitudes; do I have stereotypic perceptions?" Since disablement is a state with which most people are not intimately acquainted, it is understandable that many people have preconceived concepts regarding disabled individuals. To help clarify your attitudes toward persons with disabilities, sit back and consider: If I were to become blind, deaf, or spinal-cord injured (paraplegic in a wheelchair), how would this affect my life? Aspects of your life to consider are housing, occupation, transportation, recreational pursuits, finances, sexual function, and relationships with significant others. Could you continue your education, and if so, what modifications would be needed? Sudden adult-onset disability can impact every aspect of an individual's life. How would a disabling condition impact yours?

The impact of a disability is the perceived loss. Consider two case studies. BB is a 32-year-old married male with two young daughters. He lives in a small town and had just finished building a split-level home when he sustained a spinal cord injury due to an industrial accident. He was employed as a logger. His disability is paraplegia with complete loss of function of his lower extremities. CF is a 30-year-old single male renting a house in a large city. He is employed as a certified public accountant. He sustained a spinal cord injury due to a motor vehicle accident. His disability is also paraplegia with complete loss of function to the lower extremities. Both individuals have sustained similar loss of function. Both had a period of medical treatment and assessment. However, the perceived and realistic loss for BB is much greater. The impact of his disability affected his occupation, housing, and the relationship with his wife and children. CF returned to his previous job with the same company and moved into an accessible apartment. The adjustment for CF was much easier.

Stages of Disability
Obviously, the response to disability varies with each individual. A popular theory states that the adjustment to disability entails the individual expressing stages of anger, grief, denial, and depression. While it is true that some individuals experience such stages, it is also noted that the stages do not occur in a specific order or in a specific amount of time, and not all people experience them.

Fordyce developed a learning model with three stages to sequence the issues, which applies to adult-onset acquired disabilities.[18] The first stage, the premorbid or predisability stage, describes the temporarily able-bodied population. That's you. You have a fairly good idea of your skill level, have evaluated and chosen an occupation, recreational pursuits, and so on. You have your act together.

The second stage is the acute, or crisis, stage. With some persons this is the trauma of an accident, with others it may be the diagnosis of a major chronic disabling condition. The impact is a sudden and perhaps massive change in the individual's situation. If the individual is in the hospital, there is probably a marked decrease in pleasant events: a loss of privacy, probably physical discomfort, significant others are seen on a time contingency basis, and normal routines are disrupted. In other words, the individual has lost control over his life. Add to this a permanent disabling condition which may impact life goals, vocation, recreation, sexual functioning, and relationships with significant others. It is understandable that persons react to this situation by denial, depression, and anger.

Rehabilitation is the third stage. This is the acquisition and maintenance of behavior appropriate to the individual's new state. Because severe disability can impact all aspects of an individual's life, the adjustment or rehabilitation stage constitutes the reevaluation and learning of appropriate new behaviors which increase functioning to the maximum level possible. The patients you will be seeing will primarily be in the later stage of rehabilitation.

GENERAL MANAGEMENT CONSIDERATIONS

With any dental professional–patient relationship, the more fully you understand your patient and his psychosocial milieu and the greater awareness you have of your own attitude towards the patient, the more successful will be the treatment outcome for that patient. This holds particularly true for the patient with a disability.

If you have just been informed that your next patient is disabled but you have not yet become acquainted or seen his history, what, if any, general inferences could you safely make about the patient? You will already at this stage know several important facts. You know, for example, that your patient is a human being who—like all other people—is a distinct and unique person. As such, your patient will wish to be treated with the dignity, respect, and professional demeanor accorded all patients in your practice. At the same time, he or she would expect tactful consideration and sensitivity shown for his/her special needs.

In addition to the specific disabling condition, the patient will present with the general encumbrances which that condition has placed on his existence. The various attitudinal, physical, economic, and social problems which the patient may be experiencing may significantly affect the patient's ability to partake in dental treatment. It is essential, therefore, that you take these superimposed burdens fully into account in your problem plan and treatment for the patient.

Given this basic understanding you will feel much more competent to treat the patient with a disability, for it then becomes relatively simple to adapt your normal procedures to any special needs the patient may have. In making such accommodations the following general guidelines are helpful.

Scheduling

Appointments must be carefully planned so that maximum usage of time is made. A visit to the dental office may pose major problems for the disabled person. The patient may be coming from a considerable distance, and any special modes of transportation such as cabulances will entail additional expenses. If the patient requires the assistance of an accompanying family member or friend, arrangements may be further complicated. The dental visit may place a severe strain on the patient as well as on the companion, both of whom may have limited energy levels.

In making the dental appointment, consideration should be given to the time of day which is convenient for the patient or at which he functions best. This will vary according to the disability. For example, if Mr. Brown is a quadriplegic, your eight o'clock time slot may not allow him time to complete his bowel and bladder routine (this may take several hours), get dressed, and travel leisurely to your office. On the other hand, you will want to avoid the last appointment in the afternoon, because by that time he may be tired and so will you. For Mr. Brown, a mid- to late-morning appointment is probably most suitable. In contrast, for Ms. Smith, who is brain injured, an eight o'clock appointment may be appropriate because she is able to attend to tasks and her memory may be better earlier in the morning.

The length of the appointment may also need to be modified. In the case of Mr. Brown, it will be governed by his skin tolerance, which will determine the length of time he can sit in the dental chair. Dental treatment may need to be interrupted to allow Mr. Brown to do pressure releases, which is a method to prevent decubiti (decubitus ulcers/skin breakdown).

The best source of information on the most appropriate length and time of appointment is the patient. Do not hesitate to ask!

Physical Accommodation

The vast majority of disabled persons can be treated routinely in the ordinary dental office. Special equipment is generally not required, since most patients who are wheelchair-bound can be safely transferred to the dental chair. Once in the chair, inquire whether simple aids such as pillows or safety straps may make the patient feel more comfortable and secure.

A slight rearrangement of the reception area and hallway furniture may make the office more accessible and safer for the disabled patient. Thus, if Mrs. Black, who is legally blind and ambulates with a cane, comes to you for an examination, can she maneuver to the receptionist's desk and to the operatory without bumping into sharp-edged furniture, hanging lamps, and protruding clothes hooks? She will also be very appreciative if you adjust the light intensity to an appropriate level of comfort. Again, your best source of information is your patient. Feel free to ask.

An important point to remember is that, prior to helping a disabled individual, always inquire whether assistance is needed and how you can help. As an example, if you see an individual who is ambulating with crutches and has begun the process of opening a heavy door into your clinic, first ask "May I help you?" or "May I be of assistance?" If the individual says "Yes," then ask "How can I help?" It may be obvious that the door needs to be opened. However, the body mechanics of the individual may involve using the door as a brace and the unexpected opening of that brace may cause the individual to fall. One patient explained the process by stating, "I realize I look very awkward when getting on and off buses; however, I usually have everything under control. When I receive well-intended assistance, usually from someone behind me, I almost always fall on my face."

Treatment Planning and Consent to Care

Our professional obligation to patients is to provide the highest quality of care commensurate with the given circumstances. Any treatment plan must be realistic and may need to be modified from the "ideal" in accordance with the patient's oral condition, systemic health, and economic situation. In the dentist's judgment, the care recommended to the patient should be no less than is needed, nor more than is necessary for good dental care.[21]

It is becoming increasingly important in dental practice to ensure that the patient is fully informed of the treatment recommended, including cost; that he is fully informed of the alternatives to treatment, including nontreatment; and that the patient, after exercising his choice, gives written consent to the plan of care decided upon.

In order to be valid, such informed consent must be signed by the patient, or, if the patient is not competent to make the decision, by the legal guardian. In case of the latter, a determination of guardianship must be made. One should not automatically assume that the parent is the guardian.

The majority of retarded persons are only mildly retarded and are considered responsible for themselves. These patients must be informed in simple language which they can understand. Whether a mentally deficient or confused patient is, in fact, competent to make a decision on treatment in a given situation is left to the judgement of the dentist and depends in part on the seriousness of treatment and the associated risk factors. For example, Bill Green is a 30-year-old mildly retarded man who lives on his own with a chore worker and is legally responsible for himself. If all the treatment Bill requires is a prophylaxis and several simple restorations, Bill can safely be considered capable of giving consent. However, if Bill should need more extensive treatment such as oral surgery, entailing irreversible consequences or greater risk, it would be prudent, in addition to Bill's own consent, to obtain the written agreement also of Bill's closest relative or advocate.

Communication

In Chapter 2, the basic characteristics of facilitative communication are defined as warmth, empathy, and respect. These essential ingredients of any satisfactory dentist–patient relationship are of paramount importance in establishing rapport with the disabled patient. From the dental management perspective it is usually not the disabling condition as such, but rather the overlying functional difficulties, which create a challenge for the dentist and the entire dental team. Many difficulties can be reduced or avoided if appropriate means of communication, both verbal and nonverbal, are used and the patient's confidence gained thereby.

For the disabled patient, the basic principles of communication are equally applicable but may require some modification depending on the disability. Certainly, communication need not be verbal to convey a message. A smile or a friendly touch on the arm are signs of good will and appreciation which are part of a body language that is universally understood.

In order to be effective, communication must be at a level the patient can understand; it should neither underestimate nor overestimate the patient's intellectual capacity. Thus, if Mr. Baker has severe cerebral palsy and has great difficulty in articulation, it would be a serious mistake for you to assume that he is retarded; he might just be of above normal intelligence, working on his doctorate in engineering! In this case, you may incorrectly underestimate the patient's intellectual ability. On the other hand, even though your retarded patient may be an adult, physically and chronologically, but you know from his medical history that he is functioning at a level of a six-year-old child, you will need to communicate with him as you would with a child that age.

Communication may be difficult for both you and the patient, in that the patient may be expending considerable amounts of energy in communicating and you may have difficulty in understanding. Many times it is easier for a parent or person accompanying the patient to understand the speech patterns. However, you should always ask permission of the mentally competent patient before including another person in the interview or treatment plan process.

A modifying factor, therefore, in communicating with the disabled patient is the fact that a third party may be involved with the patient's care and welfare. This person may be a parent, an attendant, a case worker at an agency, an interpreter, or a guide. Depending on the particular situation, the dentist must then communicate appropriately not only with the patient but also with the patient's advocate or aide. Again, a good rule of thumb is that if the patient is mentally competent and responsible for himself, communicate directly with the patient. For example, 20-year-old Jane Smith, a sophomore at college who is profoundly deaf, comes to your office for an examination and prophylaxis. She is accompanied by her interpreter. The correct approach for you is to talk directly to Jane, as if the interpreter were not present. Ask Jane directly about her medical history, preference on appointments, and the like. Similarly, direct your instructions to Jane herself, not to her interpreter.

As discussed in the section on attitudes, anger and depression are emotional states which may be associated with the condition of being disabled. However, it must also be recognized that the disabled individual has the right to be angry and depressed about the same frustrations as every able-bodied person. Your patient's particular reaction may, therefore, be unrelated to the disability.

In view of the multiple problems and not infrequent confusion or limited comprehension experienced by disabled persons, it becomes all the more important that misunderstandings and unnecessary frustrations be avoided. It is best therefore, to be explicit in your communication with the patient or responsible person. Keep information simple and provide written instructions in language the patient or attendant can understand. As with all patients, detailed chart entries are a must.

The Patient's Family

The importance of the families cannot be overemphasized. In the case of a child with disability, the care and support of the child is in many cases provided solely by the family members. Because of the primary role of parents in the care of their children, there must be cooperation between parents and the health care provider. The following are guidelines in building a good relationship with the parents.

- The parents must feel that the health care provider is working with them, not against them and that together they are seeking solutions to the problems.
- The parents must feel that the health care provider likes the child and sees him/her as an individual.
- The parents must feel that the health care provider appreciates their strengths and their struggles to do the best for their child, and even though they may have shortcomings, they should not be picked on or be made to feel rejected.[20]

In the case of a sudden adult onset, it is also often the family which must provide the necessary personal care and support. This can have a great impact upon the family structure due to the amount of personal care needed by the severely disabled person. The family faces the same range of adjustment as the disabled individual; for example, families of traumatic victims also experience the three stages of Fordyce's learning model. Independent living centers are beginning to provide information and training to help the severely disabled person evaluate living style options.

A major focus in all rehabilitation centers is training disabled individuals to instruct others in their personal care. This applies also to oral hygiene. While working with the adult disabled population, especially if home care procedures are performed by a family member or attendant, it is easy but inappropriate to reduce the disabled person's responsibility for his/her dental care. The individual with the disability should assume responsibility for training others in the daily tasks of oral hygiene.

The disability of one family member places an enormous strain on the entire family. As has been pointed out, families also experience various phases of adjustment to the disability. Expressions of anger, frustration, and depression are therefore by no means limited to the patient but may be exhibited by the other persons concerned with the patient's care. The dental staff must be alert to their manifestation and recognize the underlying causes.

Managing Anxiety and Fear

Causative factors and management of dental fears, anxiety, and pain are covered in detail in the chapters devoted to these topics. Similar methods pertain to the control of anxiety in disabled patients in whom the complex interactions of fear, anxiety, and pain may be compounded by the physical and emotional problems engendered by the disability. The techniques of behavior modification and hypnosis are used very effectively with selected disabled patients. The specific modality of anxiety and pain control must be determined on the basis of the patient's condition and the dentist's preferences and experience.

In the case of the patient with a disability, it is particularly important that a calm atmosphere prevail and that stress levels be kept to a minimum for both your patient and yourself. Not only will an anxiety-free environment allow you to provide the quality of care the patient deserves and at the same time build up your own confidence, but it will prevent or minimize many untoward reactions the disabled patient might otherwise exhibit. A few examples will serve to illustrate the potentially deleterious effects of anxiety and fear.

- Anxiety is a recognized triggering factor in seizures. Not infrequently, the only time an epileptic patient experiences a seizure is shortly before a dental or medical appointment.
- Anxiety also tends to aggravate uncontrolled movements, as in a person with cerebral palsy or high-level spinal cord injury. Conversely, the more relaxed the person, the less the tendency for such movements and the easier dental management of the patient becomes.
- In a number of systemic conditions, specifically asthma, diabetes, and cardiovascular disease, the avoidance of stress becomes critical in preventing an aggravation of the disease and its symptoms.

Fear and anxiety may be the predominant features in the dental behavior of the patient who is emotionally unstable or who is mentally retarded. In fact, extensive fear may cause such patients to avoid the situation altogether; broken appointments are a common sign of their anxiety. By definition, mental retardation refers to significantly subaverage general intellectual functioning existing concurrently with deficits in adaptive behavior. To the extent that fear and anxiety can be controlled in the retarded patient, the adaptive behavior will be improved and dental management facilitated. The retarded person, when treated with respect and firmness, may in fact become an excellent dental patient who is compliant and confident.

One cause of anxiety for disabled patients which can be readily alleviated is that of fear of separation from a prosthesis or adaptive equipment. The wheelchair for the nonambulatory, the cane for the blind, or the hearing aid for the deaf become essential extensions of the disabled person's body, allowing him or her to function in the environment. An individual who uses a wheelchair and may be sitting in that wheelchair up to 14 hours per day may consider it part of his body. Leaning on it or pushing it without permission is very offensive to many individuals. One young woman who uses crutches to ambulate equates the removal of her crutches out of immediate reach with the complete loss of control. It may be impossible for an able-bodied person to understand this. However, how would you feel if, sitting in a dental chair, your legs were removed? Ridiculous! The loss of control is similar.

Always ask the patient for permission before taking adaptive equipment away, and then place it in a safe place as close to the patient as possible. If the patient cannot view it, inform him of the location.

The Team Approach

In caring for the dental patient with a disability, the value of an effective team effort becomes very evident. The team approach applies not only to full utilization of the dental staff, but must extend to other disciplines in the health care and social service fields.

In the dental area itself, auxiliaries play a vital role in the delivery of care to the disabled patient. Oral hygiene is clearly a major problem for many disabled persons and the dental hygienist may need to devise special methods of helping the patient to achieve better home care. The dental assistant also has several important functions. The assistant usually is the first person to establish contact with the disabled patient either in the office or by telephone and thus sets the tone for the entire dental experience; he/she can be a valuable aide chairside in patient management; it is frequently the assistant's task to act as a liaison with other support services, to institute referrals, and act on patient follow-up.

As with any patient, a comprehensive medical history is essential before dental treatment is performed. Since many disabled patients have serious medical problems, often entailing multiple medications, and the patient may be unable to provide a reliable history, access to the patient's medical records and consultation with the patient's physician are frequently indicated. Remember, however, that you must first obtain the patient's consent before medical records can be released.

Disabled persons in many cases have to rely on others for assistance in the performance of routine activities of daily living. Frequently they are connected with a social service agency which serves as an advocate for their needs. If such is the case, it is advisable, after obtaining the patient's consent, to establish contact with the agency in order that your treatment plan can be coordinated with the overall care plan for the patient. There are many facets relating to treatment of the disabled patient in which a social worker can be facilitative. Typical tasks for a case worker might be counseling the patient to keep dental appointments, making arrangements for transportation, and determining the availability of financial aid for the patient's dental needs.

In your position as health care provider for a disabled patient, you may be the initial person to identify a problem of a general or psychosocial nature. By referring the patient to an appropriate source of assistance, you will be providing an important link in the chain of interdisciplinary care which the person requires.

There are numerous agencies, both local and national, some of which have a specific focus (Spina Bifida, United Cerebral Palsy, Multiple Sclerosis Society, Muscular Dystrophy Association, Association for Retarded Citizens are but a few examples); others are more generalized. For the developmentally disabled, a federally mandated Protection and Advocacy System (P & A) has been established in every state for the purpose of helping disabled persons obtain needed services.

Each community develops its own information and referral system. The local office of United Way, Easter Seals, Association for Retarded Citizens, or the Crisis Clinic might be productive sources of information on available services for your disabled patient.

CONCERNING SPECIFIC DISABLING CONDITIONS

In the preceding sections, several examples have been cited of common characteristics of patients with various disabilities, apropos of dental care. The principle features of categories of disabling conditions are of concern to the dental team. It is not within the scope of this chapter to present all aspects of every disability but rather to discuss from the behavioral perspective some of the major conditions which the dentist and his or her staff are likely to encounter and some practical approaches to patient management. For a more detailed treatise of dental practice for disabled patients, the reader is referred to the available publications on this topic. A resource list of written and audiovisual materials on dentistry for the handicapped has been compiled by the American Dental Association in cooperation with the Academy of Dentistry for the Handicapped and the National Foundation of Dentistry for the Handicapped.*

* *1726 Champa, Suite 422, Denver, Colorado 80202*

The Developmentally Disabled Patient

Developmental disabilities encompass a range of conditions, principally mental retardation, cerebral palsy, epilepsy, autism, and other permanent neurological deficits which are acquired before the age of 18 years.

Mental Retardation   The mentally retarded patient is sometimes perceived by the dentist as a management problem—this patient may not sit still, may cry or make a scene, may not want dental treatment, may pose formidable difficulties in home care instruction. Yet nearly every potential problem can be avoided by good communication and a treatment plan that takes the patient's disabilities into consideration.[22]

Mental retardation is not a disease entity of itself but is a symptom of a central nervous system disorder. It rarely occurs as the only symptom and can be associated with physical and psychological abnormalities such as epilepsy, cerebral palsy, orofacial deformities, and emotional problems. Most of the retarded patients you will encounter (89 percent) will be mildly affected. Within this majority are many whose degree of retardation is so slight that, once out of school, they are functionally "normal"—they work, raise families, and lead independent lives. A smaller percentage (six percent) will be moderately retarded. The remainder (four and a half percent) comprises people in the categories of severe and profound retardation who are more likely to remain institutionalized. Depending on the degree of mental retardation and the absence or presence of other disabilities, the patient will be limited in functional capabilities.

Teaching a mentally retarded patient physical skills, such as brushing, or more abstract skills, such as nutrition, requires accurate assessment of the patient's abilities and a teaching method which takes those abilities into account.

The person with an I.Q. of 50-70 (mild retardation) can learn simple skills in great detail, but has a shorter than normal attention span and memory and lower ability to deal in abstractions. For this type of patient, you should make explanations and demonstrations short and simple and teach activities rather than concepts. Praise and reward the patient for progress made (a pat on the hand, verbal encouragement, or giving the toothbrush as a gift are effective rewards).

For the person with an I.Q. of 36-50 (moderate retardation), functional abilities will be more limited and learning will be slower; every step should be rewarded. It is best to teach those skills which the patient can successfully accomplish.

An extra effort made in communicating with your mentally retarded patient will allow him or her to develop a sense of trust and will help make the treatment experience a satisfactory one. Good rapport can be achieved in a number of ways:

- Help the patient become familiar with the dental office before treatment begins. During the first few visits you can do much to dissipate your patient's anxiety about the unfamiliar. Introduce your patient to the staff at your office; help him remember people and objects from the last visit.
- Allow yourself and your staff extra time to become familiar with your patient. This will help reduce your own anxiety about the patient.
- The first few appointments should be short, comfortable, and nonthreatening, and should not include restorative procedures.
- Give explanations slowly—at the level of the patient's mental age.
- Give only one instruction at a time. Wait to see if the patient can accomplish each step before going on to the next. For example, you may normally give a patient a series of instructions at once—to be seated, put his head back and open his mouth—with a number of explanations—that this is an exam, and so on. However, such instructions will only confuse a mentally retarded patient. Make each statement as simple and brief as possible and allow time for the patient to comply before repeating or going on.
- Make sure your patient understands you. Ask your patient to restate your instructions, either verbally or by acting them out (tilting the head back when asked, for example). "We'll have a look at your mouth now" may be clear enough to you, but your patient might respond better to a more accurate explanation and a simple instruction: "I want to look at your teeth and gums. Tilt your head back; now open your mouth."
- Reward the patient clearly and often for correct behavior. You might wish to reward your patient the way you reward your child patients, or give some other appropriate small token or reward.
- Pay attention to what your patient may be trying to tell you. Your patient may not only have trouble understanding your communications about procedures, he may also have difficulty expressing himself—even about the amount of pain being experienced. The patient's parent or attendant may be helpful in alerting you to signs that your patient is frightened, restless, or in pain, or that he wants to say something.
- In general, the Tell-Show-Do technique may be very effective in patient management.

In spite of your best efforts, you may experience management difficulties with your patient, so that treatment is deferred past the time that is necessary, convenient, or economical. For many dentists, this point is reached at the third or fourth appointment. Problems may occur for many reasons which you cannot control, as, for instance, a past traumatic experience with dentistry that has left the patient hostile to treatment. In this case, you may wish to consider pretreatment oral sedation, IV sedation, or, as a last resort, hospitalization with general anesthesia.

Cerebral Palsy Once you become familiar with the main types of cerebral palsy, you can provide the necessary contact and support which will allow you to treat most persons with cerebral palsy routinely in your office.[23]

Cerebral palsy (CP) is a broad term used to describe a group of nonprogressive disorders caused by brain damage that occurred before the central nervous system reached maturity. In addition to motor dysfunction, the cerebral palsy patient may have learning difficulties, psychological problems, sensory defects, convulsive and behavioral disorders of organic origin. While approximately 50 percent of persons afflicted with CP are also retarded, you should not assume that your patient is not of average or above average intelligence.

Uncontrolled movements tend to be the major problem in dental treatment. The best way to prevent abnormal responses or "primitive reflexes" in your patient is to determine in advance whether he usually has such responses; you can gain the requisite information from your patient, his attendant, therapist, or physician. Stimuli most likely to trigger abnormal responses are sudden noises, bright lights, abrupt changes in position, quick movements by someone in the room, or dental instruments near or in the mouth. It will be helpful to desensitize the patient gradually to these stimuli. For example, the patient with an exaggerated gag reflex could be asked to hold the mirror and move it around the mouth for a while before you attempt to do the same thing.

A quiet and relaxed atmosphere will reduce the likelihood of severe reflexes occurring. Surprises should be avoided. It is important that you tell your patient in advance when you want to change the chair position; then do it slowly. If severe responses do occur, your reassurance and kindness will be extremely helpful to your patient.

Sensory Disabilities

In treating the patient who has a severe hearing or visual impairment, good communication skills are the overriding management concern. Of the two sensory losses, deafness, while not as obvious, is formidable in the sense of social isolation and is therefore a major handicap comparable to, or more serious than, blindness.[24]

The Deaf Patient The degree of adjustment and level of achievement relate directly to individual communication skills. A patient who has had primarily positive experiences is likely to acquire an adequate sense of self-worth, security, and confidence, and these attributes will influence the patient's ability to cope with new situations such as the dental appointment. Conversely, the patient whose experiences have been basically negative will have a low self-concept and will be less able to cope with the dental experience.[24]

Time of onset of the hearing deficit plays an important role in language and personality development. In the person with congenital deafness, speech comprehension and ability will be affected, whereas if deafness is sustained after five years of age, normal language patterns tend to be maintained.

Although lack of hearing is sometimes accompanied by lack of speech, speechlessness may be a matter of individual choice. Many deaf people know that their speech patterns may cause a negative reaction in the listener and are exceedingly shy about using their voices with strangers such as the new dentist. The term "deaf-mute" is therefore very inappropriate and considered offensive.

Speech which at first seems unintelligible may be understandable to a careful listener whose own feelings do not hinder comprehension. If, however, you cannot understand the deaf patient's speech, feel free to offer pencil and paper. If the patient's writing is not standard English, it does not imply that the deaf person has less than normal intelligence. The patient may be using the grammatical structure of Ameslan (American Sign Language) which differs from that of standard English.

In communicating with your deaf patient, you may employ speech, gestures, demonstrations, sign language, written notes, or use the services of an interpreter. If the patient lip reads, use a normal voice and do not exaggerate mouth movements. Since in this situation the speaker's face rather than the patient's face needs to be illuminated, you may need to turn the operatory light off while explaining a procedure.

It is estimated that even experienced lip readers comprehend no more than 50 percent of the spoken word. You would, therefore, be well advised to use an interpreter for those phases of treatment for which accurate exchange of information is critical, such as eliciting a medical/dental history and presenting the treatment plan. Since the patient may feel self-conscious about discussing treatment in front of a close relative or friend, you must exercise tact; it might be preferable under these circumstances to use an interpreter who is less closely related to the patient.

The Blind Patient   The dentist or hygienist will find a wide variation in degree of visual impairment and will need to modify patient approach accordingly. As with other disabilities, those who are blind from birth experience blindness as an integral part of their mental and emotional growth. Those who become blind later in life are faced with the task of integrating blindness into personalities developed while still sighted.[24]

Certainly, blind individuals are as different from each other as seeing people. It is useful however, to note some common mannerisms:

- A blind person can perceive a new experience readily if it is described verbally in detail.
- The blind person has usually made an effort to cultivate the other senses such as hearing and relies on them heavily.

- A blind person will do things deliberately and slowly to gain perception and prevent accidents.
- He or she usually prefers orderliness; if something is put down, it must be readily located again.

Meeting the blind patient is much like meeting any other patient, but you may wish to take a little more initiative than usual.

- Make your presence known with an appropriate greeting and then identify yourself right away.
- If you wish to shake hands, reach for the hand even though you may need to go more than half way.
- Physical contact gives the blind person concrete evidence of your presence and replaces the customary nod or friendly smile which cannot be seen.

Do not assume that all blind people are helpless, hard of hearing, either gifted or defective, or accomplished musicians! Therefore, resist the tendency to raise your voice or to talk down to the blind person. If a sighted companion is present, do not communicate through the companion. Words like "look" and "see" are perfectly acceptable; there are no reasonable substitutes.

In guiding the blind patient, determine first what assistance, if any, he or she wants. If you imagine yourself in the patient's position, common sense and sensitivity will prevail. Usually the blind patient will have a greater sense of security and direction if he holds on to your arm just above the elbow. Inform your companion of any obstacles in your path, such as doors, stairs, curbs, and be sure to give essential details (whether the steps go up or down and how many). Giving directions by the signs of the clock is explicit (for example, "There is a chair at two o'clock ahead of you."), whereas the usual site references of "here" or "there" are meaningless to the blind person. Remember also that your patient will not be able to pick up other visual cues such as when to end a conversation; you must substitute verbal signals.

Once the patient is seated, a verbal orientation to the operatory is helpful. Be sure to introduce other personnel present and inform the patient if you leave the room. In general, avoid surprises. The patient will appreciate being forewarned of the procedure you are about to perform, whether it be the use of air, water, handpiece, or repositioning the chair.

Spinal Cord Injury

Dentistry for the spinal cord injury patient has the potential for being among the most rewarding experiences available to the dental professional. These patients may present with special problems requiring imaginative and creative solutions. Further, the oral cavity has special functional importance for high lesion quadriplegic patients. This may be the only area of their body over which they have full volitional control. The teeth and oral musculature must consequently provide the means for performing activities of daily living that would normally be accomplished by other parts of the body.[25] Helping to maintain the integrity of the dentition may add immeasurably to restoring a sense of self-worth for these patients.

The spinal cord injured patient will be all too conscious of his lost functions and may have special concerns over and above the usual dental fears, particularly in relation to transfers in and out of the wheelchair. Let the patient be your guide in how he wishes to be handled, what assistance he would like, and how he would be most comfortable. Assess the patient's psychological state, including the patient's desire for independently performing self-care tasks during the appointment (i.e., removing a sweater or detaching the wheelchair safety belt). Patients with limited muscular coordination will often indicate that they want to perform these minor tasks and "hovering" over the patient is impolite and unnecessary.

In treating the spinal cord injured patient, you must give special consideration to complicating factors which may be serious to the point of being life threatening. Such complications include decubitus ulcers (pressure sores) and dysreflexia. This is an area in which good communication with the patient is essential in order to identify potential problems and take appropriate countermeasures.

Ask the patient about his skin tolerance and how frequently he must do pressure releases. If the patient sits too long in one position, skin breakdown may occur and may cause the patient to be confined to bed or be hospitalized for weeks or even months. An existing decubitus ulcer is a contraindication to dental treatment.

Ask the patient whether he uses a catheter or external urinary collecting device. If such is the case it is important that the device is functioning properly, since an overextended bladder is the most common cause of dysreflexia—a state of acute hypertension in which the blood pressure may rise rapidly up to or beyond 300/160.

Ask the patient how he is feeling. A headache, plugged nose, and sweating forehead are signs or symptoms of dysreflexia. The patient may also experience other discomforts which might be alleviated through appropriate positioning or supports. Each patient should be able to direct his care to avoid serious complications.

Stroke

Stroke, or cerebrovascular accident (CVA), is the third leading cause of death in the United States. The stroke patient you see in your private practice possibly will be one of your regular patients, and it may be difficult for you both to adjust to the severe changes that the patient suddenly manifests;

a formerly active, gregarious person may have difficulty finding words and be totally dependent on others. Management of the stroke patient will depend largely on the extent of the deficit and functional capabilities remaining.[26]

If the stroke occurred on the left side (right hemiplegia), speech and language ability may be impaired. Deprived of the capacity to communicate, such a patient may become bewildered, frustrated, and angry when interaction with others proves difficult. The right hemiplegic tends to be anxious, slow, and disorganized. Simple, frequent feedback will help this patient to learn or relearn oral health habits; demonstration is preferable to verbal instruction. Even though he cannot use speech, this patient's ability to learn and communicate should not be underestimated.

The stroke patient with right brain damage (left hemiplegia) may have difficulty with spatial–perceptual tasks and have impaired judgment. Because this patient can communicate, it is easy to overestimate his abilities. Verbal instructions are best, but the patient should demonstrate that he can perform a given task.

In patient management, the dentist must be aware of other common physical and behavioral sequelae of stroke.

- Brain function on one side may be impaired; the patient may be paralyzed and have visual field cuts. He may not see or respond to people, objects, or events on the impaired side.
- The patient may neglect the impaired side even to the point of not recognizing the impaired side as part of his body.
- The patient may exhibit personality changes. A formerly fastidious, compliant patient may be sloppy, irritated, or uncooperative.
- The patient may have an impaired memory, particularly for recent events, and decreased visual and/or auditory retention. He may have difficulty carrying skills learned in one environment over to another.
- The patient may be emotionally labile (i.e., may cry frequently, laugh inappropriately, have flare-ups of temper or sullenness). Such emotional changes may be the result either of depression or of damage to the brain as the result of the stroke.
- The patient may exhibit sensory deprivation and as a result be susceptible to sensory overload.

In view of the deficits incurred, a number of management strategies are indicated in the dental situation.

- Always stand on the patient's "good" side; present objects and demonstrations to this side.
- Provide instruction and information in short, simple segments. A "re-

minder" list to post in the bathroom will help to orient the patient to home care tasks.

- Interrupting emotional behavior due to brain damage will help the patient avoid embarrassing or fatiguing activity and may be accomplished by snapping your fingers or calling the patient's name.
- Minimize distractions in the office. Scheduling the patient for a time when the waiting room is not crowded or turning the dental chair so that the patient's "good" side faces a quiet area of the room are simple ways of eliminating extraneous stimuli.

By helping disabled people to achieve good oral health, you will add an important dimension to their lives. An attractive smile, a functioning dentition, and the knowledge that you, as a dentist, care, will add substantially to the person's self-esteem; in turn, it will have a positive effect on how others perceive that individual. You will find that kindness and understanding will go a long way in establishing a trust relationship with the patient, enabling you to accomplish the necessary dental care. In the process, you will earn not only the gratitude of the disabled patient and the patient's family, but you will also gain much personal satisfaction.

REFERENCES

1. Snow, M.; Hale, J. M.; Stiefel, D. J. *Disabled Dental Patients—How Many?* Seattle, Washington, Project DECŌD, School of Dentistry, University of Washington, 1978.
2. Public Law 93-516, 93rd Congress, H.R. 17503, December 7, 1974, *Rehabilitation Act Amendments of 1974.*
3. Dunham, J. R. and Dunham, C. S. "Psychosocial aspects of disability." In *Disability and Rehabilitation Handbook,* edited by R. M. Goldenson, J. R. Dunham, C. S. Dunham. New York: McGraw-Hill, 1978, pp. 12–14.
4. Public Law 93-112, 93rd Congress, H.R. 8070, September 26, 1973, *Rehabilitation Act of 1973.*
5. Nowak, A. J. "Dental care for the handicapped patient—past, present, future." In *Dentistry for the Handicapped Patient,* edited by A. J. Nowak. St. Louis: C. V. Mosby, 1976.
6. Swallow, J. N. and Swallow, B. G. "Dentistry for physically handicapped children in the international year of the child." *Internat Dent J* 30:1, 1980.
7. Brown, J. P. "The efficacy and economy of comprehensive dental care for handicapped children." *Internat Dent J* 30:14, 1980.
8. Bureau of Economic & Behavioral Research, American Dental Association. *Profile of the Disabled Population in the United States,* Chicago, 1979.
9. Stiefel, D. J.; Lubin, J. H.; Truelove, E. L. "A survey of perceived oral health needs of homebound patients." *J Pub Health Dent* 39:7, 1979.

10. Kamen, S. "History of dentistry for the handicapped: past, present and future." *Canad Dent A J* 7:347, 1976.
11. Bentz, G. H.; Lotzkar, S.; Alcorn, B. C.; Barber, T. K.; Bystrom, E. B.; Henson, J. L.; Plummer, M. W.; Simon, J. F.; Stiefel, D. J. (A Joint Committee of The American Association of Dental Schools and the National Foundation of Dentistry for the Handicapped). "Curriculum guidelines in dentistry for the handicapped: National Conference on Dental Care for Handicapped Americans/Education Programs in Dentistry for the Handicapped." *J Dent Educ,* Part 2 of 2, September, 1979.
12. Roberts, R. E.; McCrory, O. F.; Glasser, J. H.; Askew, C. Jr. "Dental care for handicapped children reexamined: Dental training and treatment of the handicapped." *J Pub Health Dent* 38:22, 1978.
13. U.S. Department of Health, Education and Welfare, Public Health Service. *Specialized Training for Dentists Treating Children with Handicaps: An Evaluation.* DHEW Publication No. 78-5218 Washington, D.C.: Government Printing Office, 1978, pp. 94–101, 113–115, 119–121.
14. Kinne, R. D. and Stiefel, D. J. "Assessment of student attitude and confidence in a program of dental education in care of the disabled." *J Dent Educ* 43:271, 1979.
15. Gellman, W. "Roots of prejudice against the handicapped." *J Rehab* 25:4, 1959.
16. Zola, I. K. Personal communication, 1977.
17. Mitchell, J. and Allen, H. "Perception of a physically disabled counselor in a counseling session." *J Counsl Psychol* 22:70, 1975.
18. Sayer, A. E. "Social attitudes of university students toward the disabled: Contributory factors." *Am A Rehab Therapy J* 26:26, 1978.
19. Fordyce, W. E. "Behavioral methods in rehabilitation." In *Rehabilitation Psychology,* edited by W. Neff. Washington, D.C.: American Psychological Assn., 1971.
20. Wright, B. A. *Physical Disability: A Psychological Approach.* New York: Harper & Row, 1960
21. Gurney, N. L. and Alcorn, B. C. "The concept of attitudes." In *Dentistry for the Handicapped Patient,* edited by K. E. Wessels. Postgraduate Dental Handbook Series, Vol. 5. Littleton, Mass.: PSG Publishing Company.
22. Snow, M. K. and Stiefel, D. J. *Dental Treatment of the Mentally Retarded Patient.* Seattle, Wash. Project DECŌD, University of Washington, 1978.
23. Danforth, H. A.; Snow, M.; Stiefel, D. J. *Dental Management of the Cerebral Palsied Patient.* Seattle, Wash. Project DECŌD, University of Washington, 1978.
24. Engar, R. C. and Stiefel, D. J. *Dental Treatment of the Sensory Impaired Patient.* Seattle, Wash. Project DECŌD, School of Dentistry, University of Washington, 1977.
25. Schubert, M. M.; Snow, M.; Stiefel, D. J. *Dental Treatment of the Spinal Cord Injured Patient.* Seattle, Wash. Project DECŌD, School of Dentistry, University of Washington, 1977.
26. Schubert, M. M.; Snow, M. K.; Stiefel, D. J.; DeFreece, A. *Dental Treatment of the Stroke Patient.* Seattle, Wash. Project DECŌD, School of Dentistry, University of Washington, 1978.

10

Oral Habit Disorders

JOHN D. RUGH AND J. WILLIAM ROBBINS

Much of clinical dentistry is involved with modifying structural aspects of the stomatognathic system. Placing a three-unit bridge, delivering a lower denture, or endodontically treating a tooth are procedures to improve structural aspects of the oral cavity. The suitability and longevity of these structural corrections, however, depends upon the patient's oral behaviors (i.e., what he or she does with the mouth). Just as the successful periodontal surgery will depend upon the patient's oral hygiene, the success of a new denture or a three-unit bridge often depends upon the oral motor behaviors of the patient. The most meticulous dental work can be destroyed in a few months' time through self-destructive oral habits such as nocturnal bruxism, daily clenching, or abnormal postural habits (See Fig. 10-1). Such self-destructive oral habits can also have a deleterious effect upon oral soft tissue. Many cases of muscular pain and tenderness, muscular hypertrophy, periodontal tissue injury, ligament damage, and disc disorders have been attributed to persistent or forceful oral habits. Self-destructive oral habits are believed responsible for a large percentage of the dentist's problem cases. It is thus essential that the dentist be able to identify and manage problematic oral habits. The purpose of this chapter is to present information which will help you understand the etiology and characteristics of various harmful oral habits and to be aware of procedures to identify and manage these problems.

This chapter is not intended to serve as a comprehensive literature review. Rather, it is a synthesis of clinical impressions and research. Its purpose is to introduce the problem of oral habits and provide practical methods of identifying and managing these problems.

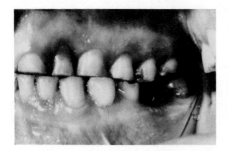 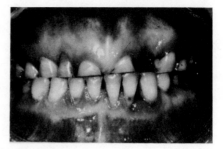

FIG. 10-1. Tooth wear from nocturnal or daytime bruxism may have occurred during a stressful period in the patient's life several years ago. Alterna-
tively, the patient may still be an active grinder. The advisability of starting
extensive restorative procedures depends upon determining the patient's
current oral habit situation.

DAYTIME ORAL HABITS

Daytime oral habits include teeth clenching and grinding, cheek and tongue
biting, finger and thumbsucking, unusual postural habits, unilateral chewing, and a wide range of habits related to the patient's occupation. Habits
such as thumbsucking are more common among children while others,
such as abnormal postural habits, are more common among adults. In most
cases, the effects of oral habits are minimal and transitory; however, they
can also be problematic. Daytime oral habits have been suggested as etiological factors in malocclusion, tooth wear, speech and swallowing difficulties, periodontal disease, denture soreness, mandibular dysfunction, and de-
struction of expensive restorative efforts.[1]

Incidence and Etiology

Some oral habits such as thumbsucking are common. It is reported that over
half the children, during infancy or childhood, suck their thumbs.[2] If
thumbsucking is stopped by age four or five, the effects are generally insig-
nificant. However, thumbsucking past the age of five may result in elonga-
tion of the anterior segment of the maxillary arch, Class II malocclusions,
and narrowing of the maxillary arch. Children who suck past the age of six
seldom have normal occlusion.[3] One study[4] has reported that thumbsucking is greater among girls than boys.

Historically, it was believed that oral habits were manifestations of serious unconscious emotional disturbances. Psychoanalytically oriented therapists recommended that these problems should be treated by attending to
the underlying psychopathology. This view is no longer widely held. While
oral habits may accompany certain emotional difficulties, there is no evidence that the emotional disorder will intensify by treating the self-destruc-

tive oral habit. There have been numerous psychological studies of patients suffering from masticatory symptoms believed related to oral habits. These patients were found by various investigators to be perfectionists, hypernormal, responsible, aggressive, obsessive, anxious, and sometimes hypochondriacal.[5] However, there is little evidence to suggest that most TMJ or MPD patients suffer from serious psychopathology, treatable only through psychotherapy.

Daytime oral habits may be best understood in terms of learning principles.[6] Most human behavioral patterns are acquired through learning. Both normal and abnormal behavior are governed by specific stimulus conditions or by the consequences of the behavior. Thumbsucking in the child, for example, may be reinforced by the attention it brings from the parent. Although the attention may be in the form of a reprimand, many children find any attention preferable to none at all. Other oral behaviors may be reinforced through chance pairing with a reinforcing event. For example, chewing on a pencil during a test may be reinforced by the solution to a test question. Except for a few innate and reflexive functions, most human oral behaviors are governed by their consequences. Attention to this important principle is essential in the understanding and management of oral habits.

Unusual postural habits which exemplify learning principles have been noted by orthodontists. A habitual maintenance of a protruded mandibular posture is common in patients with a retrognathic mandible. The patient learns to compensate for the "weak jaw" by holding the mandible forward. This requires continuous activity of the lateral pterygoid muscles and sometimes results in muscle tenderness or pain. Patients are often unaware of the habit. It becomes a postural position which is automatic after the initial learning. Such overlearned automatic postural habits are often very difficult to alter (See Fig. 10-2).

Increased tension in muscles and changes in mandibular posture have been found to accompany emotional states such as anxiety, frustration, or

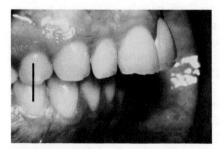 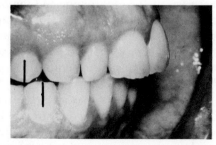

FIG. 10-2. Patients with a retrognathic mandible often learn to compensate for the "weak jaw" by holding the mandible forward. This postural position may become automatic and result in muscle fatigue and tenderness.

fear.[5,7] When emotional pressures are prolonged or intense, muscular pain or tenderness can result. Patients with myofascial pain symptoms commonly present with histories of other psychophysiological complaints such as low back or neck pain, ulcers, nervous stomach, and asthma.[8] Questioning of these patients often reveals that their presenting oral symptoms are only one aspect of a broader set of somatic stress-related symptoms. Over 50 percent of the 135 MPD patients evaluated by Gold, et al.[8] were frequent users of psychotropic medication. This suggests that the oral symptoms may be only one aspect of a more general psychophysiological disorder. The dentist must evaluate the patient's emotional conditions and oral habits carefully before concluding that the symptoms are due to a local stimulus such as an occlusal prematurity. In many cases, mandibular dysfunction symptoms are the result of muscular tension and emotional stress.[9] A thorough history is the best guide to differentiate between occlusal and emotional etiologies.

Altered oral function can also result from time pressures. When subjects are forced to rush through a meal, as is common in our hurried western lifestyle, masticatory function may be dramatically altered. Rugh[10] reported that when subjects are rushed through a meal, they chew faster, with greater force, and with fewer pauses between bursts of chewing. These changes are accompanied by a reduction in the number of chewing strokes per volume of food ingested. The significant increases in force and changes in the timing of the chewing strokes may contribute to masticatory dysfunction and fractures of teeth.

The etiology of some oral habits and muscle hyperactivity is iatrogenic. Dentures with increased vertical dimension may elicit increased masticatory muscle activity and oral habits. It is common for muscle activity to increase slightly when a new denture is inserted. The initial discomfort in wearing the prosthesis often results in an increase in muscular activity (See Fig. 10-3). Zarb[11] has noted that the complaint of a sore tongue is frequently related to the habit of thrusting the tongue against the new denture. As with many oral habits, the patient is usually unaware of the causal relationship between the painful tongue and the habit. Zarb has also noted that patients tend to occlude the teeth often at first to "test" the new denture. This hyperactivity associated with adaptation is probably normal. However, if the muscle hyperactivity and mucosal soreness continue, the dentist should carefully reevaluate the denture, the patient's emotional situation, and oral habits.

In most cases of masticatory dysfunction, the problem is multifactorial (i.e., the patient may have a stress-related teeth clenching problem, malocclusion, and TMJ arthritis). The challenge is usually not to determine which etiological factor is involved but rather to what degree each factor is involved. Not only must the structural features of the oral cavity be evaluated, but the patient's emotional condition must also be carefully examined. In

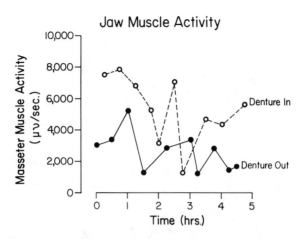

FIG. 10-3. Muscle hyperactivity resulting from a denture with increased vertical beyond an acceptable level is demonstrated in this 48-year-old female patient. Muscle activity generally doubled with the denture in the mouth. Muscle activity and pain symptoms were relieved through remaking dentures with a 5 mm decrease in vertical dimension.

addition, it is important to check for oral habits and to question the patient regarding recent lifestyle changes of major life events which may influence the patient's oral health.

Identification of Daytime Oral Habits

Identification of self-destructive oral habits may include the use of questionnaires, patient interviews, and daily pain charts. Electromyographic recording may also be used in the clinic and in the patient's home to help identify problem oral behaviors. The first goal is to identify the habit and demonstrate its relation to the patient's problem. Next, stimuli which elicit or maintain the habit must be identified. An intelligent treatment strategy can be selected only with such etiological knowledge. For example, treatment for a teeth clenching habit which results from an occlusal irritation may be managed through occlusal adjustment. However, a similar habit in another patient may be caused by strenuous physical effort (See Fig. 10-4). Many individuals find that they clench their teeth when performing a physical task. An occlusal adjustment in this latter case would be of little value in eliminating the habit. Progressive relaxation and learning differential control of muscle groups would be more appropriate therapies. Likewise, teeth clenching in a patient attempting to hold in a maxillary removable appliance which has poor retention may be stopped by improving the retention of the appliance. The stimuli or conditions which maintain the habit must be identified to select a logical therapeutic approach.

A self-administered questionnaire regarding the patient's oral habits

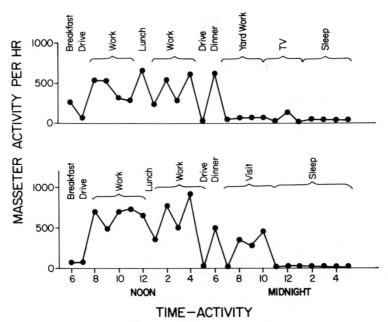

FIG. 10-4. Electromyographic recording of the masseter over a two-day period in a 52-year-old male presenting with muscular pain, fatigue, and excessive tooth wear. These recordings indicated intense muscular contractions associated primarily with work. Muscle activity during his work hours was equivalent to that used during eating. Muscle activity was minimal during sleep, suggesting no nocturnal bruxism. The patient's symptoms were relieved through habit retraining.

(Figure 10-5) may be a routine aspect of the patient's intake procedure. It should be part of the patient's permanent record and may provide you with clues in finding a solution to a difficult treatment situation. You should review the questionnaire and ask the patient to expand on items marked "yes." A number of problems can be identified with this tool. The questionnaire also serves to document oral habits which in the future may cause other oral dysfunction.

Questionnaires are economical in that they reduce patient–doctor contact time; however, they must not be seen as a substitute for the chairside history. The patient should be given ample time and encouragement to express concerns and problems. The questioning need not be heavily structured; rather it should be casual and open. It may begin with questions about the patient's current oral symptoms and gradually move to queries regarding family situations, employment, economic and medical problems. An in-depth psychiatric evaluation is not usually necessary to understand a patient's stress problems or identify a problematic oral habit.

Patient _____ Date _____

PATIENT QUESTIONNAIRE

	Yes	No
1. Do you clench or grind your teeth during the daytime? (Specify when)	___	___
2. Has anyone heard you grinding in your sleep?	___	___
3. Have you awakened with your teeth tightly clenched?	___	___
4. Are pain symptoms more severe upon waking?	___	___
5. Do your teeth, gums, or muscles feel sore when awakening in the A.M.?	___	___
6. Have you recently (2 months) had a major change in your lifestyle, marital status, employment, or other matters which you feel are important?	___	___
7. Do you chew on objects (pencils, finger nails, etc.)?	___	___
8. Does gum chewing or eating big meals leave your jaw sore or tired?	___	___
9. Do you chew on your lip, tongue, or cheek?	___	___
10. Do you chew mostly on one side?	___	___
11. Do you clench your teeth when angered, frightened, bored, or frustrated?	___	___
12. Has a recent accident, dental procedure, or other event called attention to your mouth?	___	___
13. Do you now take tranquilizers?	___	___
14. Do you now have or have you had a history of ulcers, spastic colon, skin ailments, hypertension, hyperventilation, tachycardia, tension head or neck aches or other disorders which may be related to stress?	___	___
15. What does the pain you are experiencing keep you from doing, i.e., how has your problem altered your lifestyle?		

FIG. 10-5. Self-administered questionnaire may be filled out by the patient in the waiting room. The dentist should review the questionnaire with the patient and discuss, in depth, those questions marked "Yes."

A valuable tool to help identify the etiology of some myofascial pain symptoms is the patient hourly pain chart, such as that shown in Figure 10-6. Pain charting serves several functions. First, it provides valuable diagnostic information regarding the frequency, timing, and intensity of the patient's symptoms which often helps identify the origin of the pain. Daily or weekly cycles are frequently apparent and provide clues to etiology. The pain records should be discussed with the patient and an attempt made to identify relationships between pain cycles and changes or events in the patient's life. The records frequently make it easy to demonstrate to the patient the relationship between stress, muscular habits, and pain. Often, daily pain records must be made over one or two months to identify cyclic problems. A major advantage of the pain chart is that it involves the patient in the solution of the problem. The patient recognizes that the solution to symptoms may rely upon changing behavioral patterns or lifestyle.

Portable electromyographic biofeedback devices may be useful in help-

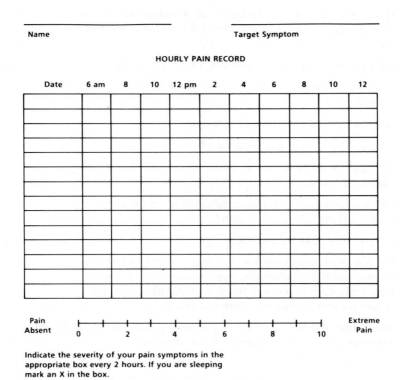

FIG. 10-6. Hourly pain records filled out by the patient over a two-week period often show trends in the patient's condition which help pinpoint the etiology of the patient's problem.

ing to identify and stop some teeth clenching habits. The portable EMG instrument provides a tone in the patient's ear when tooth clenching occurs.
This technique calls attention to the clenching and allows the patient to
identify stressful situations which are related to the clenching. Often patients are unaware of their oral habits. The portable EMG device allows the
patient to report precisely what habits are involved and exactly how they
are performed (i.e., which teeth are touching, how the mandible was positioned, and situations which elicit the habit). Frequently, patients can learn
to control the habit in one or two days when it is brought to their attention
in this manner. Solberg and Rugh[12] reported that ten of 15 patients using a
portable signaling device showed clinical improvement in their facial pain
symptoms. These patients were able to identify stimuli which caused their
clenching and grinding. All 15 patients were surprised to find how frequently they clenched and believed they benefited by this insight.

Cigarette smoking is perhaps the most insidious of oral habits. The relationship of smoking to cancer, heart disease, and emphysema is often discussed; however, Solomon, Priove, and Bross[13] noted that many smokers
show greater concern with the prospect of periodontal disease or tooth loss
than the prospect of lung cancer or heart disease. Evidence has been presented indicating that both men and women who smoke cigarettes have a
higher prevalence of periodontal disease.[13,14] The oral cavity of a smoker
may show a grayish discoloration and leukoplakia of the soft tissue. A
brown discoloration of tooth surfaces is sometimes accompanied with tar-
like deposits. The health hazards associated with smoking are well known in
the United States and smoking is becoming less socially acceptable. Bumper
stickers reading "kissing a smoker is like licking an ash tray" express the
distaste some have for the habit. The outlook for a reversal in the smoking
habits of the American public, however, is not optimistic. Advertising by
the tobacco companies will likely prevail over warnings of the medical, dental, and governmental agencies. Recent statistics indicate that smoking
among males has leveled off at about 37.5 percent. Smoking among females,
however, has been steadily climbing coincident with massive cigarette advertising campaigns launched toward females.

As a dentist, you can play a role in helping the smoker to reconsider the
advisability of this oral habit. Many of the hazards of smoking are long
range and not salient to the patient. Short-term effects, however, can be
shown in the oral cavity. Using a mirror, you can show the patient the teeth
staining and the tissue changes. This demonstration coupled with a brief
explanation of the relationship between smoking, periodontal disease, and
tooth loss may contribute to the smoker's decision to quit.

Overzealous oral hygiene and abuse of toothpicks may also result in
damage to oral structures. Ideally, these instruments remove plaque and
massage the gingiva; however, if used improperly, patients may present

with gingival recession and abrasion of the teeth. The gingival margin is often enlarged or "piled up" and large interproximal spaces may be observed where debris may collect. Aggressive brushing is often found in individuals who are perfectionists. They engage in toothbrushing like many other activities with the belief that a little is good and more is better. Usually the problem of excessive or improper brushing is easily corrected by a brief explanation of the problem. Patients who brush excessively are generally eager to please and correct such undesirable behavior. Habitual use of toothpicks is less easy to alter. Toothpicks can be used in almost any environment and patients report that the stimulation of the tissue provides a pleasant sensation; something similar to scratching a mosquito bite. With these patients, a more forceful and stronger argument must be presented. This may include showing the patient the damage, discussing the significance of the damage, and suggesting an alternative habit which may be less damaging yet provide oral stimulation. Gum chewing may be a more suitable habit.

Teeth may be loosened, intruded, and tilted by a variety of objects placed in the mouth. Musical instruments may place prolonged or excessive pressure against the teeth, resulting in migration or periodontal injury. Likewise, the mouthpiece of the scuba diver and other objects related to occupation placed in the oral cavity must be suspect when evaluating the patient's oral condition. Query the patient about objects which are commonly placed in the mouth. Noting these in the patient's record may serve to explain the etiology of later problems.

Management of Daytime Oral Habits

Daytime oral habits have been treated in a variety of ways. When muscle pain is involved, immediate temporary relief of symptoms may be accomplished by a combination of Fluori-Methane spray, tranquilizers, heat packs, muscle exercises, aspirin, and soft food diet. If the patient is anxious or fearful about the condition, the first step in therapy is to relieve the fears and anxiety. Explain the problem to the patient in simple terms. It is important to indicate to the patient that the condition is not unique. The patient is not suffering some unusual or unknown disorder.

The selection of a method for long-term management of oral habits and associated symptoms depends upon the precise nature of the habit and the patient's motivation and intelligence. When compliance or patient motivation is a problem, mechanical appliances which prevent the habit are useful. Intraoral appliances are ideal in children or in adults who seem unwilling to make conscious efforts to help themselves. The palatal crib, for example, has been shown to be very effective in stopping thumbsucking (See Fig. 10-7).[15] Its use requires only minimal effort on the part of the patient. Likewise, an occlusal splint used to manage daytime teeth clenching

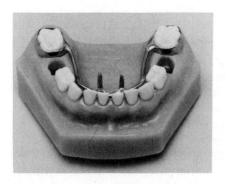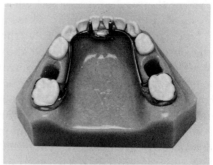

FIG. 10-7. A lower arch appliance designed to alter swallowing patterns, reduce thumbsucking, and help correct anterior open bites *(from Williams & Lecocq, 1980).*

requires little effort on the part of the patient and provides excellent clinical results.[16] Although a palatal crib has been shown to be effective in stopping thumbsucking, such mechanical restraint has not been found effective in permanently altering tongue thrust swallowing. Subtelny and Subtelny[17] report that even after six months of treatment with a tongue crib, tongue thrusting returned within three months after treatment. Recently, Williams and Lecocq[18] have experimented with a mandibular crib which warrants testing. Disadvantages of all mechanical forms of therapy are their side effects. Both the splint and the palatal crib disrupt speech and normal swallowing patterns and susceptibility to caries is increased with their use. Finally, many patients are concerned about the aesthetics of wearing these appliances.

When patient compliance and motivation are not a problem, other forms of therapy which have fewer side effects may be used. A variety of exercises have been developed which are designed to increase the patient's awareness of a specific habit and eventually control it. Such self-control procedures are all that are required to break many self-destructive oral habits.

One self-control exercise to increase awareness of a habit involves the patient purposely practicing the habit in front of a mirror. The patient must attend carefully to the proprioceptive feelings related to the habit. It is believed that the exercise increases the patient's ability to recognize the occurrences of the habit and thus allows the control of it. Another method of habit management requires that the patient keep a record of the habit occurrences. Finally, portable EMG devices are useful in increasing patient awareness of oral habits and in providing a means to control these habits.

As public education regarding the side effects and morbidity associated with drugs and other treatment modes increases, there will be more patients who are skeptical of drugs and who are unwilling to put up with the side effects of intraoral appliances. These patients feel responsible for their health and are generally eager to involve themselves in self-control therapies. The self-control therapies mentioned above are ideally suited for these patients.

There exists considerable controversy over the etiology and management of some oral problems. Tongue thrust swallowing is a case in point.[19] Tongue thrusting was believed to be an etiological factor in anterior open bite. Furthermore, it was held that orthodontic correction of the open bite would fail if the deviate swallowing patterns were not treated. An elaborate treatment program called "Myofunctional Therapy" was developed and thousands of clinicians have been trained in the procedures. When myofunctional therapy is used, the success rate in modifying a swallow is 70 to 80 percent. However, this is about the same as would be expected from spontaneous recovery due to developmental factors. The controversy over myofunctional therapy and tongue thrust swallow culminated in a Joint Committee[20] of the Representatives from the American Association of Orthodontists and the American Speech and Hearing Association. This committee reviewed relevant studies and presented a policy statement which indicated that there was no acceptable evidence to support claims of significant, stable, or long-term changes in swallowing patterns or oral form with myofunctional therapy. Well-controlled clinical studies of most therapeutic procedures are lacking, unfortunately, so claims of therapeutic effects must be cautiously evaluated.

NOCTURNAL BRUXISM

Clenching or grinding of the teeth during sleep has been reported in the earliest records of humans. Bruxism during sleep consists of two basic patterns. Rhythmic, chewinglike movements are observed which involve intense vertical and lateral pressures to the teeth. The second pattern involves intense, prolonged contractions of the muscles with the mandible in either centric occlusion or eccentric positions (See Fig. 10-8). During these periods, the masticatory muscles have been observed to remain in continuous contraction for periods of up to 300 seconds. Episodes of bruxism activity occur periodically during sleep; however, the episodes have been reported to be more frequent during early morning hours. Bruxism episodes do not usually occur while dreaming but rather when the patient is going from a deeper to a lighter stage of sleep. It is often accompanied by a change in heart rate and respiratory patterns suggesting an arousal phenomenon. A bruxism episode may be initiated by stimulating the sleeper with unusual noises or calling out the sleeper's name.[21]

In western cultures, reports on the incidence of bruxism range from 5 to 80 percent. The discrepancy in these estimates is believed to result from

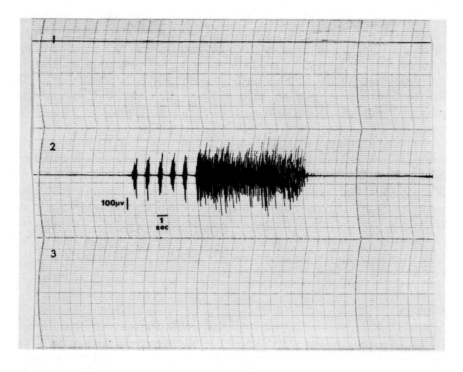

FIG. 10-8. Electrical activity of the masseter muscle of a patient during a nocturnal bruxism episode. This patient shows rhythmic contractions similar to chewing followed by a sustained maximal contraction of approximately ten seconds. Some patients have been observed to clench or grind 1200 seconds per hour of sleep. Such bruxism activity may result in muscle fatigue and pain, tooth wear, and joint pain.

the way in which bruxism is assessed. When patients are asked if they grind their teeth, only about five percent answer affirmatively.[22] However, if bruxism is evaluated through more objective means, such as tooth wear, estimates range from 50 to 80 percent.[23,24] Tooth wear can result from many oral activities and probably overestimates the incidence of bruxism. A reasonable estimate is that about 30 percent of the population exhibit nocturnal bruxism. Of this number, only a few will exhibit the behavior to the extent that it is pathologic. Mild to moderate tooth wear is found in many healthy individuals. It is believed normal and is usually ignored by most dentists. The effects of bruxism, however, are not always so benign. A number of patients will present with serious oral lesions from bruxism. Excessive abrasion may cause pain and the disruption of normal masticatory function.[25] Cases have been reported in which excessive tooth wear resulted in pulpal death.[26]

The prolonged and intense periods of muscular contraction during nocturnal bruxism are believed responsible for patient reports of muscle fatigue and tenderness upon rising. From an analysis of wear patterns, it is apparent that bruxism often involves eccentric, unstable positioning of the jaw. Pressures applied in these unstable positions are believed responsible for tooth mobility, traumatic lesions within the connective tissue of the muscles and tendons, and damage to the temporomandibular joint structures.

The incidence of bruxism is equal in males and females, although it is common to find more women seeking treatment of problems believed related to bruxism.[27,28] The reason for this is not known. Nocturnal bruxism is reported in both children and adults. Clinically, one finds children between the ages of three and 12 who exhibit grinding. Parents are often alarmed at the intensity of the grinding noises and concerned about the potential damage which might result from such insidious behavior. Most children seem to stop grinding by age 12. The damage is seldom significant and no treatment is usually indicated.

Etiology

Several theories have been suggested to account for nocturnal bruxism. A commonly held view is that occlusal discrepancies may trigger nocturnal bruxism. Historically, it was believed that the patient's nocturnal grinding was an unconscious effort to relieve an irritating occlusal discrepancy. Occlusal adjustment, or equilibration, was seen as a logical therapy. Recent investigations, however, in which nocturnal bruxism was actually measured suggest that occlusal factors have little, if anything, to do with triggering nocturnal bruxism. When high restorations are placed in patient's mouths, an increase in nocturnal bruxism has not been found.[29] Nor has it been found that occlusal adjustment reduces a patient's nocturnal clenching and grinding.[30] Although oral structural features (malocclusion) may not be a causative factor in nocturnal bruxism, it is believed that a patient with structural weakness may suffer greater consequences from bruxism. Thus, although therapy directed at occlusal discrepancies may not alter the frequency or magnitude of the patient's grinding, such therapy may strengthen the structure and limit the damage.

Current evidence suggests that nocturnal bruxism is a stress–related sleep disorder.[21,31-33] Incidences of bruxism have been closely tied to emotional stress and/or physical exhaustion during waking hours (See Fig. 10-9). Emotional stress during waking hours such as intense fear, anger, or apprehension are known to dramatically disrupt normal sleep patterns. The disruptive effects may be mediated through the chemical changes that occur in the body when stressed. It is well known that each individual responds differently to emotional stress. Some respond with increased stomach acidity and ulcers; others respond with profuse sweating, cardiac symptoms, vaso-

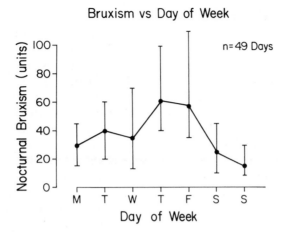

FIG. 10-9. Nocturnal bruxism is frequently related to stressful life events. Bruxism was highest in this 32-year-old female on Thursdays and Fridays when work pressures were greatest. The patient seldom ground her teeth on Sunday nights when she felt most relaxed.

constriction of the hands, muscular tension, irregular shallow breathing, or a spastic colon. Some believe that an individual's unique response to stress is learned, while others hold that it is genetically determined. There is evidence that individuals have a genetic predisposition to nocturnal bruxism;[34] however, the problem may also be stimulated by focusing attention in the oral cavity.

Although most cases of nocturnal bruxism in adults are due to emotional stress, bruxism has also been reported in some cases of brain damage and as a drug side effect. Use of amphetamines, for example, has been reported to result in nocturnal bruxism.[35] Many weight-control programs involve the use of amphetamines. Severe bruxism has also been observed in patients with tardive dyskinesia which is believed to be a complication of long-term phenothiazine usage.[36] Fenfluramine, an amphetamine derivative, has also been implicated as a causative agent in bruxism.[37] The patient should be questioned about the use of such drugs. Nocturnal bruxism accompanying brain damage is easily identified, as the patient usually displays other physical or mental disabilities.

In summary, it is believed that nocturnal bruxism is basically a stress-related sleep disorder related to emotional stress during waking hours. It may be mediated by the hormonal changes which accompany psychological or physical stress during the waking hours. Nocturnal bruxism in children may also result from a hormonal imbalance. With children, however, the hormonal imbalance may be due to a developmental problem. There is evidence that individuals may inherit a predisposition for nocturnal bruxism.

Identification of Nocturnal Bruxism

A diagnosis of nocturnal bruxism is often difficult to substantiate. Several diagnostic methods have been used with different degrees of success (See Fig. 10-10). As in all areas of dental or medical diagnosis, the patient history is of paramount importance in diagnosing nocturnal bruxism. Such questions as: "Are you aware that you grind your teeth?" or "Has anyone ever told you that you grind your teeth?" are logical introductory questions. The responses to these questions, however, must be interpreted in light of the fact that most bruxist patients are unaware of their nocturnal habits. Also, a sleeping partner will only be made aware of the activity if it involves a significant lateral component resulting in grinding noises.

Destructive clenching in eccentric jaw positions must be identified by other means. The following clinical signs and symptoms are useful in diagnosis:

- Tooth wear—Study casts are helpful in locating facets of wear. It is instructive to position the maxillary and mandibular casts such that the

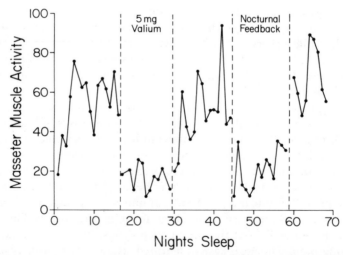

FIG. 10-10. Nocturnal bruxism may be suppressed for short periods through administration of 5 mg Valium 30 minutes before bedtime or through sounding a tone with each bruxism event (Nocturnal EMG Feedback). Either method may be useful to assist in identifying the etiology of the patient's facial pain symptoms. This patient's muscle fatigue and unilateral temporal pain were eliminated when grinding was reduced through Valium (days 17–29) and nocturnal biofeedback (days 45–58). The bruxism and symptoms returned when treatment was stopped (days 60–68).

wear facets are aligned. This often involves an eccentric positioning of the mandible. The instability of this position often helps explain the nature of the subject's joint, ligament, and muscular symptoms.

- Tooth mobility—Tooth mobility is not singularly diagnostic of bruxism. However, in the absence of other etiologies such as advanced periodontal disease, mobility is a reliable indication of parafunction.
- Fractured teeth—Vertical fractures and fractured cusps may indicate bruxist activity.
- Muscle tenderness—Palpation of the muscles of mastication is helpful but not totally reliable in diagnosing nocturnal bruxism.
- Muscle hypertrophy—Patients with a long-standing history of bruxism classically have enlarged masseter muscles.
- Headache—Headache in the temporal area often accompanies nocturnal bruxism. Patients will frequently report a pulling sensation in the temporal muscle region.

A diagnosis of nocturnal bruxism may be strengthened by the diagnostic administration of 5 mg diazepam (Valium) before bedtime for one week. Diazepam appears to reduce bruxism.[33] The patient should report a dramatic reduction in symptoms upon the next visit. The same logic is used with the application of short-term nocturnal EMG biofeedback. Nocturnal bruxism can be sharply reduced if the subject is aroused by a tone when the event occurs. Symptoms related to the behavior should be significantly reduced within a few days. The clinician must always keep in mind that nocturnal bruxism is highly variable from night to night. It may disappear for weeks or months but reappear as stressful life events are encountered.

Management of Nocturnal Bruxism

Treatments used to manage nocturnal bruxism fall into three categories. These are psychological, structural, and pharmacological. None of the treatments have been found to be 100 percent effective nor to permanently stop nocturnal bruxism. Grinding and clenching during sleep persistently tracks the patient's emotional lifestyle; bruxism will increase under times of stress then subside during periods of calm. The symptoms related to bruxism may be relieved temporarily through drugs, an occlusal splint, or nocturnal biofeedback. Long-term management of the problem, however, typically requires the patient to alter his or her lifestyle to reduce stress. Nocturnal bruxism is seldom cured; rather, the problem must be continuously "managed." Since it is so closely linked to the patient's lifestyle, the ultimate responsibility for the problem must lie with the patient.

Any approach to therapy should start with an explanation of the etiology of the problem. The probable etiology of nocturnal bruxism should be explained to the patient in simple, nontechnical terms. Analogies may be made to commonly understood stress-related disorders such as ulcers or tension headaches. The patient should understand that the problem is a manifestation of a chosen lifestyle and that the ultimate responsibility for the problem is in the patient's hands (See Fig. 10-11). This should be presented carefully in a nonthreatening and nonjudgmental manner. Indicate to the patient that the disorder is not an indication of a mental disorder but typically results from the pressures of daily life. Express concern for the patient's general health, prior stress-related problems, and the pressures of modern lifestyle. (Most dentists can show empathy with patients having stress-related problems, as they often have first-hand experience with such

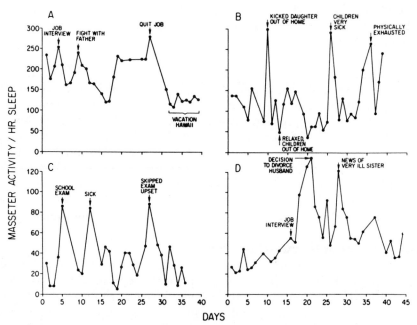

FIG. 10-11. Nocturnal bruxism of four patients demonstrating the relationship of nocturnal bruxism to life events. Treatment of Patient A whose bruxism is chronic may be with long-term splint usage or a comprehensive stress control program. Patients B and C who brux only periodically may be managed by short-term counseling. Patient D whose bruxism was related to an infrequent life event (divorce) may have been best managed by short-term (two-week) use of tranquilizers given during the peak of her emotional difficulties. Appropriate treatment of the bruxist patients depends upon the nature of the problem. This information can normally be obtained through a careful history taking. (*From Rugh, J. D. and Solberg, W. K. Electromyographic studies of bruxist behavior before and after treatment. Calif. Dent A J 3:56, 1975.*)

problems.) The advantages and limitations of various treatments for nocturnal bruxism are discussed briefly below.

Pharmacological Management   Oral administration of centrally acting sedatives (5 mg. Valium) 30 minutes before the patient retires is effective in relieving nocturnal bruxism and related symptoms for short periods of time. Increased dosages are required with prolonged usage and for this reason, long-term drug therapy is discouraged. Pharmacological management is indicated where the patient's stress is identified as being self-limiting and recovery is expected. Nocturnal bruxism and emotional distress resulting from a divorce, death in the family, or unusual financial crisis would be expected to reach a peak, then dissipate. Drug therapy may be a treatment of choice in these cases.

Occlusal Splint (Nightguard)   Splint therapy remains the most effective method for management of symptoms related to nocturnal bruxism regardless of etiology.[38] Symptom improvement can be expected in 80 to 90 percent of the cases even though nocturnal EMG studies indicate that only about one-half of the subjects actually show a reduction in bruxism.[16] Thus, although many subjects will continue to grind and clench on a splint, their symptoms are relieved. This is probably the result of the redistribution of forces. Use of the splint is indicated where the symptoms have persisted for prolonged periods, where there is danger of destroying reconstructive work, where the patient is incapable of or unwilling to accept counseling, or where occlusal factors are salient.

Occlusal Adjustment   Since occlusal prematurities have been considered by many to be the primary etiologic agent in bruxism, occlusal adjustment has often been used to treat the problem. Many claim success in occlusal treatment, especially in alleviating muscle pain secondary to muscle hyperactivity.[39]

General Stress Control Program   A comprehensive program designed to alter dramatically the patient's lifestyle is the treatment of choice. It may include counseling, biofeedback, progressive relaxation, hypnosis, dietary evaluation, change in occupational status, and other methods. Several programs include the teaching of coping skills. Stress control programs are ideal for individuals whose general mental health is fine but who have a history of other stress-related disorders and who recognize the need to alter their lifestyle. Stress control programs have been developed in numerous clinics throughout the United States in recent years. Patient response to these programs has been excellent.

Psychotherapy   Extensive psychological counseling may be required where nocturnal bruxism appears as a component of major psychological disturbances. Construction of a nightguard is usually indicated in these cases to protect the patient during the period of psychological therapy. Nocturnal biofeedback is not indicated in these cases as the patients are seldom in condition to take advantage of such self-help strategies.

A number of other therapies have been used with nocturnal bruxism. These include a "massed practice" procedure where the patient intentionally clenches during the day, auto suggestion, hypnosis, and dietary supplements. There is little evidence that these methods significantly alter nocturnal bruxism.[30,32]

The selection of an appropriate therapy will be greatly aided by a careful review of the patient's recent history and current lifestyle. When emotional or physical stress are factors, it must be established during the patient history whether the situation is expected to be short term or chronic. Also determine if the patient has other stress-related problems and recognizes the need to alter his or her lifestyle. Attention to the emotional needs and lifestyle of patients greatly enhances the probability of selecting a satisfactory therapeutic approach.

Assessment of Therapy

The therapist must periodically assess the efficacy of management of the bruxist or oral habit patient and make adjustments in therapy as indicated. Assessment, however, is difficult and often misleading for several reasons. First, the musculoskeletal pain symptoms related to oral habits (nocturnal and diurnal) are commonly cyclic and self-limiting in nature. Over a period of months, the symptoms often intensify, peak, and then decrease. The cycle will frequently repeat itself with some exacerbations being more severe than others. The difficulty lies in the fact that patients usually report for help when the symptoms are at a peak. Anything the doctor does is likely to be followed by a reduction in symptoms. It is extremely difficult to determine if the symptom relief was due to the therapy or the cyclic nature of the disorder.

A major problem in assessing the effect of treatment is the lack of the patient's awareness of the behavior. With respect to nocturnal bruxism, the reports of a sleeping partner are often difficult to interpret. The sleeping partner's assessment of bruxism usually depends upon being awakened by the noises of grinding. The assessment may thus depend more upon the quality of the partner's sleep rather than the degree of the bruxist's activity.

Accurate assessments of nocturnal bruxism have been made using portable EMG instruments which record electrical activity of the patient's masseter muscle in the home. Another assessment procedure involves indexing the degree of bruxism by evaluating wear patterns on laminated acrylic sheets vacuformed on a study model to fit over the patient's teeth. Unfortunately, these assessment procedures are available only in a few university clinics. At this time, assessment must rely primarily upon the patient's complaints and history, as well as the clinical examination.

Treatment strategies for oral habit disorders should begin with conservative, reversible procedures such as counseling, biofeedback, minor sedatives, and occlusal splints. Escalation of therapy to nonreversible therapies such as occlusal adjustment should be made with considerable caution. The possibility of developing an occlusal neurosis in an emotionally unstable patient must be carefully evaluated.

Prognosis and Referrals

The number of patients seeking treatment for oral habit disorders has increased steadily during the last two decades. As a dentist, you have responsibility for diagnosis and treatment of oral conditions, including those related to oral habits. The majority of self-destructive oral habits and their related symptoms can be successfully managed in the dental office through structural changes, pharmacological therapy, or brief counseling. There are, however, patients whose oral habit behavior or emotional problems are not easily managed. You can be emotionally and financially drained by such a patient if the patient shows no improvement or becomes increasingly ill despite ideal occlusal relationships and attempts at counseling made by the dentist. Clinical experiences suggest that patients who are not likely to get well without more extensive counseling are patients who:

- Have centered their life around their pain symptoms for six months or longer. They have overreacted to relatively minor symptoms. The symptoms have become salient features of their lives.
- Receive secondary gain for the symptoms. Such patients are receiving economic and social benefits for maintaining a sick role. They may be using the symptoms to avoid social life, work, parenting, or a variety of other responsibilities.
- Report symptoms in vague, nonspecific terms. Symptoms are often presented in theoretical terms and are poorly localized.
- Have a history of several other stress-related disorders.
- Blame another dentist for initiating the current problems. These patients are frequently more interested in revenge than in finding a solution to their pain symptoms.

You may justifiably prefer to refer these patients to a mental health professional for more comprehensive counseling. However, the ideal solution to most oral habit disorders is through a team approach involving the dentist, a behavior therapist, and a motivated patient.

REFERENCES

1. Bryant, P.; Gale, E.; Rugh, J., eds. *Oral Motor Behavior: Impact on Oral Conditions and Dental Treatment*. NIH Publication #79-1845. Washington, D.C.: U.S. Government Printing Office, 1979.
2. Ayer, W. A. "Thumb-finger sucking and bruxing habits in children." In *Oral Motor Behavior: Impact on Oral Conditions and Dental Treatment,* edited by P. Bryant, E. Gale, J. Rugh. NIH publication #79-1845, 1979, pp. 7–22.
3. Popovich, F. and Thompson, G. W. "Thumb and finger-sucking; its relation to malocclusion." *Am J Ortho* 63:148, 1973.
4. Kelly, J.; Sanchez, M.; Van Kirk, L. *An Assessment of the Occlusion of Teeth of Children.* DHEW Publication NO. HRA 74-1612. National Center for Health Statistics, U.S. Public Health Service, 1973.
5. Rugh, J. D. and Solberg, W. K. "Psychological implications in temporomandibular pain and dysfunction." In *Temporomandibular Joint: Function and Dysfunction,* edited by G. Zarb and G. Carlsson. St. Louis: C.V. Mosby, 1979, pp. 240–68.
6. Bandura, A. *Principles of Behavior Modification.* New York: Holt, Rinehart & Winston, 1969.
7. Yemm, R. "Causes and effects of hyperactivity of jaw muscles." In *Oral Motor Behavior: Impact on Oral Conditions and Dental Treatment,* edited by P. Bryant, E. Gale, J. Rugh. NIH publication #79-1845, 1979, pp. 138–56.
8. Gold, S.; Lipton, J.; Marbach, J.; Gurion, B. "Sites of psychophysiological complaints in MPD patients: II. Areas remote from the orofacial region." *J Dent Res* 54(Special Issue A):165, 1975. (Abstract #480).
9. Laskin, D. M. "Etiology of the pain dysfunction syndrome." *Am Dent J A* 79:147, 1969.
10. Rugh, J. D. "Variation in human masticatory behavior under temporal constraints." *J Comp Physio Psychol* 80:169, 1972.
11. Zarb, G. A. "Oral motor behaviors and oral prostheses." In *Oral Motor Behaviors and Oral Disorders,* edited by P. Bryant, E. Gale, J. Rugh. Washington, D.C.: U.S. Government Printing Office, 1979, pp. 227–41.
12. Solberg, W. K. and Rugh, J. D. "The use of biofeedback devices in the treatment of bruxism." *S Calif Dent A J* 40:852, 1972.
13. Solomon, H. A.; Priove, R. L.; Bross, I. D. "Cigarette smoking and periodontal disease." *Am Dent A J* 77:1081, 1968.
14. Schwartz, D. M. and Baumhammers, A. "Smoking and periodontal disease." *Perio Abstract* 20:103, 1972.
15. Haryett, R. D.; Hansen, F. C.; Davidson, P. O.; Sandilands, M. L. "Chronic thumbsucking. The psychologic effects and relative effectiveness of various methods of treatment." *Am J Ortho* 53:569, 1967.
16. Clark, G. T.; Beemsterboer, P. L.; Solberg, W. K.; Rugh, J. D. "Nocturnal elec-

tromyographic evaluation of myofascial pain dysfunction in patients undergoing occlusal splint therapy." *Am Dent A J* 99:607. 1979.

17. Subtelny, J. D. and Subtelny, J. D. "Oral Habits: Studies in form, function and therapy." *Angle Ortho* 43:347, 1973.

18. Williams, T. R. and Lecocq, K. R. "A simple tongue-thrust appliance." *J Pedo* 4(4):299, 1980.

19. Mason, R. M. "Tongue thrust." In *Oral Motor Behavior: Impact on Oral Conditions and Dental Treatment,* edited by P. Bryant, E. Gale, J. Rugh. NIH Publication #79-1845, 1979, pp. 32–48.

20. Joint Committee on Dentistry and Speech Pathology. "Position statement on myofunctional therapy." *Am Speech and Hearing A J* 16:347, 1974.

21. Satoh, T. and Harada, Y. "Electrophysiological study on tooth grinding during sleep." *Electroenceph Clin Neurophysiol* 35:267, 1973.

22. Reding, G. R.; Rubright, W. C.; Zimmerman, S. O. "Incidence of bruxism." *J Dent Res* 45:1198, 1966.

23. Frölich, E. "Die Parafunktionen: Symptomatologie, Ätiologie und therapie." *Dtsch Zahnärztl Z* 21:526, 1966.

24. Leof, M. "Clamping and grinding habits, their relation to periodontal diseases." *Am Dent A J* 31:184, 1944.

25. Glaros, A. G. and Rao, S. M. "Effects of bruxism. A review of the literature." *J Prosth Dent* 38:149, 1977.

26. Ingle, J. I. "Alveolar osteoporosis and pulpal death associated with compulsive bruxism." *Oral Surg Oral Med Oral Path* 13:1371, 1960.

27. Franks, A. S. T. "The social character of temporomandibular joint dysfunction." *The Dent Pract* 15(3):94, 1964.

28. Helöe, B. and Helöe, L. A. "Characteristics of a group of patients with temporomandibular joint disorders." *Com Dent Oral Epid* 3:72, 1975.

29. Barghi, N.; Rugh, J.; Drago, C. "Experimentally induced occlusal dysharmonies, nocturnal bruxism and MPD." *J Dent Res* 58(Special Issue A):316, 1979.

30. Bailey, J. O. Jr. and Rugh, J. D. "Behavioral management of functional oral disorders." In *Oral Motor Behaviors and Oral Disorders,* edited by P. Bryant, E. Gale, J. Rugh. Washington, D.C.: U.S. Government Printing Office, 1979, pp. 160–78.

31. Clark, G. T.; Rugh, J. D.; Handelman, S. L. "Nocturnal masseter muscle activity and urinary catecholamine levels in bruxers." *J Dent Res* 59(10):1571, 1980.

32. Glaros, A. G. and Rao, S. M. "Bruxism: A critical review." *Psychol Bul* 84:767, 1977.

33. Rugh, J. D. and Solberg, W. K. "Electromyographic studies of bruxist behavior before and after treatment." *Calif Dent A J* 3:56, 1975.

34. Abe, K. and Shimakawa, M. "Genetic and developmental aspects of sleep-talking and teeth-grinding." *Acta Paedopsychiatrica* 33:339, 1966.

35. Ashcroft, G. W.; Eccleston, D.; Waddell, J. L. "Recognition of amphetamine addicts." *Brit Med J* 1:57, 1965.

36. Kamen, S. "Tardive dyskinesia, a significant syndrome for geriatric dentistry." *Oral Surg Oral Med Oral Path* 39:52, 1975.

37. Brandon, S. "Unusual effects of fenfluramine." *Brit Med J* 4:557, 1969.

38. Zarb, G. A. and Speck, J. E. "The treatment of mandibular dysfunction." In

Temporomandibular Joint: Function and Dysfunction, edited by G. Zarb and G. Carlsson. St. Louis: C.V. Mosby, 1979.

39. Ramfjord, S. P. "Dysfunctional temporomandibular joint and muscle pain." *J Prosth Dent* 11:353, 1961.
40. Bailey, J. O. Jr. and Rugh, J. D. "Effect of occlusal adjustment on bruxism as monitored by nocturnal EMG recordings." *J Dent Res* 59(Special Issue A):317, 1980.

Appendix

Instructions for Relaxation Training and Systematic Desensitization

PROGRESSIVE RELAXATION TRAINING

Progressive relaxation training consists of a series of exercises in which a muscle group is alternately tensed and relaxed. The patient is first instructed to produce tension in a specific muscle group by, for example, clenching his fist. Tension is maintained for approximately ten seconds, during which the instructor points out the discomfort associated with tension and helps the patient focus his attention on these sensations.

The patient is then instructed to relax the muscle group as completely as possible, letting the tension dissipate abruptly rather than gradually. During this 20 second period of relaxation, the instructor points out the comfortable feelings associated with relaxation and helps the patient focus his attention on these sensations.

The tension–relaxation cycle is repeated for the same muscle group before proceeding to the next muscle group in the series. Typically, 16 muscle groups are covered sequentially in this fashion.

We have found it useful to vary speech rates for tension and relaxation instructions. For example, the word "Now" is spoken sharply when it is a signal to produce tension. During the ten-second tension period, the instructor speaks at a normal rate. The words "Now relax" signal the onset of the 20-second relaxation period and are said in a soft tone. During the relaxation period, the instructor speaks slowly and in a monotonous, soothing tone.

Relaxation instructions are presented below. Phrases in italic are instructions to the instructor and should not be read to the patient.

Instructions for Progressive Relaxation

Lean back in the chair and get as comfortable as you can. (*Five-second pause*) Close your eyes and let your body relax as you sink down into the chair. (*Five-second pause*) Take a deep breath, then exhale slowly. As you exhale let your body sink deeper into the chair. (*Ten-second pause*)

I will ask you to tense, then relax, various muscles in your body. As you tense one group of muscles, try to keep the rest of your body relaxed. We will begin with your right hand.

1. *Right Hand*
   a. *Tension* (*ten seconds*) When I say "Now," clench your right fist tightly. Remember to keep the rest of your body relaxed. Now! Clench your right fist. Feel the tension in your fingers and your knuckles. Notice how uncomfortable this feels. Pay attention to the tension in your hand, your fingers and your arm. (*Continue for remainder of ten-second interval*)
   b. *Relaxation* (*20 seconds*) Now relax. Let go of the tension in your hand. Let go completely and all at once. Let your hand and your fingers and your arm become loose and limp. Notice how much more comfortable your hand and arm feel when they are relaxed. Let the tension continue to drain down your arm and out through your fingers. Let the tension flow out and away and let the relaxation take over. (*Continue for remainder of 20-second interval*)
   c. *Repeat a and b above*
2. *Right Arm*
   a. *Tension* (*ten seconds*) When I say "Now," tense the biceps in your right arm by pushing your right elbow down against the chair. Remember to keep the rest of your body relaxed. Now! Push your right elbow against the chair. Feel the tension all through your arm. The muscles in your arm feel stiff and tense and uncomfortable. Concentrate on the tension all through your arm. (*Continue for remainder of ten second interval*)
   b. *Relaxation* (*20 seconds*) Now relax. Relax and let go of all the tension in your arm. Let the tension flow away and let your arm become loose and limp. Imagine that your arm is like an old piece of rope that has been tossed on the ground—completely limp, no tension anywhere. Let your hand and your arm become heavy and let them sink into the chair. (*Continue for remainder of 20-second interval*)
   c. *Repeat a and b above*

3. *Left Hand*
    a. *Tension (ten seconds)* When I say "Now," clench your left fist tightly. Now! Clench your left fist and notice how tense and uncomfortable you feel. Focus on these unpleasant sensations. The muscles in your left hand and arm feel tight and uncomfortable. (*Continue for remainder of ten second interval*)
    b. *Relaxation (20 seconds)* Now relax. Let the tension flow out and away from your hand and your arm and your fingers. Let your arm become limp and heavy and let it sink down into the chair. Notice the difference between tension and relaxation. Pay attention to the comfortable feeling of relaxation. Continue to let your hand and your arm relax further and further. (*Continue for remainder of 20-second interval*)
    c. *Repeat a and b above*
4. *Left Arm*
    a. *Tension (ten seconds)* When I say "Now," tense the biceps in your left arm by pushing your left elbow down against the chair. Remember to keep the rest of your body as relaxed as possible. Now! Push your left elbow against the chair. You can feel the tension throughout your left arm and into your left hand. It feels very stiff and uncomfortable. Pay attention to these feelings of tension and stiffness. (*Continue for remainder of ten-second interval*)
    b. *Relaxation (20 seconds)* Now relax. Let go of all the tension in your hand and your arm and your fingers. Let the tension drain away and let your arm become limp and heavy. Even when you think your arm is completely relaxed, continue to let go even further. (*Continue for remainder of 20-second interval*)
    c. *Repeat a and b above*
5. *Forehead and Scalp*
    a. *Tension (ten seconds)* When I say "Now," I want you to produce tension in your forehead and scalp by raising your eyebrows as high as you can. Now! Notice how tense and uncomfortable you feel. Your forehead and scalp are tight and stiff—very uncomfortable. (*Continue tor remainder of ten-second interval*)
    b. *Relaxation (20 seconds)* Now relax. Let your eyebrows return to their normal position and let all the muscles in your scalp and around your eyes relax. Let your forehead and scalp smooth out—picture them becoming smooth as the relaxation spreads. Notice the difference as you let go of the tension in these muscles. You feel much more comfortable. (*Continue for remainder of 20-second interval*)
    c. *Repeat a and b above*
6. *Eyes, Nose*
    a. *Tension (ten seconds)* When I say "Now," squint your eyes very tightly shut and wrinkle up your nose. Now! Squint your eyes

tightly and wrinkle your nose. Tension in this area is very uncomfortable. Pay attention to these sensations. Your face feels very tight
and tense. (*Continue for remainder of ten-second interval*)

   b. *Relaxation* (*20 seconds*) Now relax. Let go of all of the tension around
your eyes and around your nose. Notice the difference between tension and relaxation. Try to turn these muscles off, as if you were
turning off a light. Continue to let the relaxation spread all across
your face and scalp. (*Continue for remainder of 20-second interval*)

   c. *Repeat a and b above*

7. *Mouth, Jaws*

   a. *Tension* (*ten seconds*) When I say "Now," clench your teeth tightly
together, pull the corners of your mouth back like a jack-o-lantern,
and press your tongue against the roof of your mouth. Now! Clench
your teeth, pull the corners of your mouth back, and press your
tongue against the roof of your mouth. This feels very uncomfortable. Pay attention to these uncomfortable sensations. (*Continue for
remainder of ten-second interval*)

   b. *Relaxation* (*20 seconds*) Now relax. Turn these muscles off. Let them
go loose and limp and let your head become very heavy. Let the
chair support your head. Notice how much more comfortable you
feel as the tension drains out and away from these muscles. Let your
head become heavier and heavier as it rests against the chair. Much
more comfortable—very calm and relaxed. (*Continue for remainder of
20-second interval*)

   c. *Repeat a and b above*

8. *Neck*

   a. *Tension* (*ten seconds*) When I say "Now," push your head back
against the chair so that you feel tension in your neck. Remember to
keep the rest of your body relaxed. Now! Feel the tension. Your
neck feels stiff and uncomfortable. Notice the unpleasant sensations
—pay close attention to them. (*Continue for remainder of ten-second interval*)

   b. *Relaxation* (*20 seconds*) Now relax. Turn these muscles off. Let them
go loose and limp and let your head become very heavy. Let the
chair support your head. Notice how much more comfortable you
feel as the tension drains out and away from these muscles. Let your
head become heavier and heavier as it rests against the chair. Much
more comfortable—very calm and relaxed. (*Continue for remainder of
20-second interval*)

   c. *Repeat a and b above*

9. *Shoulders, Upper Back*

   a. *Tension* (*ten seconds*) When I say "Now," take a deep breath hold it,
and pull your shoulder blades together in the back. Remember to
keep your arms, face, and neck relaxed. Now! Take a deep breath,

hold it, and pull your shoulder blades together. Notice how awkward and rigid this feels. Imagine holding this position for more
than a few minutes; it would become very painful. (*Continue for remainder of ten-second interval*)
  b. *Relaxation* (*20 seconds*) Now relax. let go of all the tension in these
muscles and let them become limp. Turn off these muscles completely. Let your shoulders fall naturally into place. Breathe easily
and gently and notice how much more comfortable you feel. Your
arms feel relaxed, your face, your scalp, your neck—all very relaxed, very comfortable. (*Continue for remainder of 20-second interval*)
  c. *Repeat a and b above*
10. *Abdomen*
  a. *Tension* (*ten seconds*) When I say "Now," tense the muscles in your
abdomen. Tense up as if someone were going to hit you in the stomach. Remember to keep the rest of your body relaxed. Now! Hold
these muscles tense and rigid. Notice how very tight and uncomfortable you feel. it's difficult to breathe properly—very uncomfortable, very unpleasant. (*Continue for remainder of ten-second interval*)
  b. *Relaxation* (*20 seconds*) Now relax. Let these muscles become limp
and relaxed. Notice how much easier it is to breathe. Breathe free
and easily; in and out, in and out. Each time you exhale, let these
muscles relax even further. Let your body become heavier and heavier as you sink down into relaxation. Even when you think you are
completely relaxed, continue to let go. (*Continue for remainder of 20-
second interval*)
  c. *Repeat a and b above*
11. *Right Thigh*
  a. *Tension* (*ten seconds*) When I say "Now," tense the large muscle on
top of your right thigh. Keep the rest of your body relaxed. Now!
Hold the tension in this muscle. Notice how stiff and uncomfortable
it feels. (*Continue for remainder of ten-second interval*)
  b. *Relaxation* (*20 seconds*) Now relax. Let go of the tension in this muscle and let your leg become very heavy. Let go and let your leg sink
down into the chair. Turn off these muscles and let the relaxation
proceed on its own. Notice how much more comfortable this feels.
(*Continue for remainder of 20-second interval*)
  c. *Repeat a and b above*
12. *Right Calf*
  a. *Tension* (*ten seconds*) When I say "Now," tense the muscles in your
right calf by pulling your toes up toward your head. Try to point to
your face with your toes. Now! Concentrate on the feeling of tension. Notice how stiff and rigid your leg feels. Stretch these muscles
and feel the tension. (*Continue for remainder of ten-second interval*)
  b. *Relaxation* (*20 seconds*) Now relax. Let go of the tension all at once

and turn off these muscles. Let these muscles become completely limp. Let your leg become heavy, very heavy. let it sink down into the chair as you let it become heavier and heavier. Notice how comfortable this feels. (*Continue for remainder of 20-second interval*)

   c. *Repeat a and b above*

13. *Right Foot*

   a. *Tension* (*ten seconds*) When I say "Now," point the toes on your right foot away from your face and curl them under toward the bottom of your foot. Now! Feel the tension through your foot and ankle. Notice how stiff and uncomfortable these muscles feel when you tense them. It feels very unpleasant. (*Continue for remainder of ten-second interval*)

   b. *Relaxation* (*20 seconds*) Now relax. Let your foot straighten out as these muscles are turned off. Turn the muscles off completely and let your foot become loose and limp and relaxed. Let your foot and your leg become very heavy and let them sink into the chair. Continue to let the relaxation take over. Notice how comfortable you feel. Continue to breathe easily and gently, in and out (*Continue for remainder of 20-second interval*)

   c. *Repeat a and b above*

14. *Left Thigh*

   a. *Tension* (*ten seconds*) When I say "Now," tense the large muscle on top of your left thigh. Remember to keep the rest of your body as relaxed as possible. Now! Hold the tension and notice how uncomfortable this feels. Pay attention to these sensations. Your leg feels stiff and rigid. (*Continue for remainder of ten-second interval*)

   b. *Relaxation* (*20 seconds*) Now relax. Turn off the muscles in your leg just as if you were turning off a switch. Turn off the tension. Let the tension flow out and away and let your leg sink down into relaxation. Let your leg become heavy and let it sink down into the chair. (*Continue for remainder of 20-second interval*)

   c. *Repeat a and b above*

15. *Left Calf*

   a. *Tension* (*ten seconds*) When I say "Now," tense the muscles in your left calf by pulling the toes on your left foot toward your face. Point your toes toward your face. Now! Stretch these muscles so that they're tense and rigid. Notice the uncomfortable sensations. (*Continue for remainder of ten-second interval*)

   b. *Relaxation* (*20 seconds*) Now relax. Let go of the tension in your leg, in your foot, in your toes. Let your leg become relaxed as these muscles become limp and loose. Let your leg become heavy and let it sink down into the chair. Let the tension flow out and let the relaxation take over. (*Continue for remainder of 20-second interval*)

c. *Repeat a and b above*
16. *Left Foot*
  a. *Tension (ten seconds)* When I say "Now," point the toes on your left foot away from your face and curl them under toward the bottom of your foot. Now! Focus on the tension in your left foot and your left ankle. Notice how stiff and rigid your foot and ankle feel. Focus on the difference between tension and relaxation. (*Continue for remainder of ten-second interval*)
  b. *Relaxation (20 seconds)* Now relax. Turn off the tension in these muscles and let the tension wash away, drain away from your foot and your leg. Let the relaxation take over as the tension drains away. Notice the comfortable sensations that accompany relaxation. Let your leg and your foot become very heavy. Let them sink down into the chair. (*Continue for remainder of 20-second interval*)
  c. *Repeat a and b above*

Let your body become very heavy. Let your body sink down into the chair, down into relaxation. Breathe easily and gently, in and out, in and out. Now you can sink even deeper into relaxation by taking a deep breath and exhaling very slowly. As you exhale, let your body sink down deeper into relaxation. You feel very comfortable, very calm, very peaceful. Continue to breathe quietly, calmly, in and out. Enjoy the peaceful feeling of relaxation.

FEAR HIERARCHY

Below is a sample hierarchy for fear of dentistry. After the patient has been trained in progressive muscle relaxation (this usually requires two to four office sessions, or one office session and one to two weeks of daily practice at home), the patient is instructed to relax and hierarchy items are presented sequentially.

Each item is presented for approximately ten seconds. During the ten-second presentation, the instructor continues to describe the scene as the patient visualizes it. The scene should be described in as much detail as possible as an aid to visualization.

The patient is then instructed to stop imagining the scene. He is instructed to relax and to imagine a peaceful scene, such as lying on a beach or floating on a cloud or a feather bed. Again, the instructor should describe the scene in detail during this interval, which should be about 30 seconds in duration.

The scene from the hierarchy is then presented again for ten seconds, followed by 30 seconds of relaxation. The instructor then proceeds to the next hierarchy item and so on, presenting each hierarchy item twice.

Sample Hierarchy

   1. You are calling to make a dental appointment. First, you look up the number in the telephone book. Then you dial the number and hear the telephone ring at the other end. The receptionist answers. You give your name to the receptionist and tell her that you have a tooth that has been bothering you. The receptionist gives you a choice of dates and times. You select one and make an appointment.

   2. You are driving to your dental appointment. You drive out of your neighborhood, past some familiar stores and landmarks. As you drive, you begin to think about your dental appointment. You hope the tooth won't have to come out. You feel a little uneasy, but you are pretty sure you can handle it. Now you are approaching the part of town where your dentist's office is located. You are driving slowly, looking for a parking space.

   3. You park your car. Now you are walking from the street toward the dentist's office. You enter the main door of the building and walk toward the elevator. The elevator takes you up two stories. You leave the elevator and walk down the hall to the dentist's office.

   4. You enter the waiting room. You notice the smells associated with a dentist's office. You give your name to the receptionist who smiles and asks you to have a seat. You ask if the wait will be long. The receptionist tells you that the dentist is right on schedule and will be with you in just a few minutes.

   5. You are seated in the waiting room, awaiting your turn. You pick up a magazine and leaf through it. A mother and a little boy are seated across the room from you. The mother is reading to the little boy. You watch them for a minute or two. You think about being seated in the chair with the dentist working on your teeth and you feel a little uncomfortable. You wonder what he will do. You take a deep breath and relax and figure it probably won't be all that bad.

   6. The dental assistant comes out to the waiting room and asks you to come in. The dentist is ready to see you. You follow the dental assistant who shows you to the dental chair and asks you to be seated. You sit in the chair, looking around at all the instruments. The dental assistant adjusts the chair and places a napkin around your neck.

   7. The dentist enters and says hello. You talk with him for a minute or two. He washes his hands and, drying them, sits down next to the dental chair. He asks you what brings you to his office and you tell him about the pain you've felt in a lower back tooth. He listens attentively and asks you some questions.

   8. The dentist says he would like to examine the tooth. He picks up a small mirror and a probe and asks you to open your mouth. You open your mouth. The dentist asks you to point to the tooth that has been bothering you. You point. The dentist gently probes around the tooth. You can feel the probe against your gums.

9. The dentist tells you that there is an area of decay where part of an old filling has fallen out. He tells you that he would like to remove the remainder of the old filling and the decay and fill the tooth. You feel relieved that he can save your tooth.

10. The dentist asks if you would like some anesthetic. You hesitate, then tell him that you are a little bit afraid of needles. You decide to have the anesthetic, but you feel uneasy while he is preparing the injection. You take a deep breath, close your eyes, and sink into the chair. You decide that it will be easier if you are relaxed.

11. The dentist gives you the anesthetic injection. You feel a pinch. It stings a little bit. You start to tense up, but then you remember to take a deep breath and let your body relax as much as possible. You feel a second pinch. The dentist says, "There. All finished." You decide it wasn't so bad, after all.

12. You are sitting in the chair, waiting for the anesthetic to take effect. Your mouth feels numb. The dentist checks your mouth and says he can begin. He tells you to signal him if you would like him to stop at any time. This makes you feel a little better.

13. The dentist is drilling your tooth. You hear the drill and you feel the sensation and the vibrations. It's becoming tiring, holding your mouth open. You begin to feel restless. Then you tense slightly, let go of all the tension, and relax. You begin to think about other things.

14. The dentist has finished drilling and is ready to fill your tooth. He inserts the filling material and packs it in place firmly. He works on your tooth with several instruments. You feel very bored, so you begin to think about a trip you are planning.

15. The dentist asks you to bite down gently. You bite down. He asks you to open your mouth again, makes an adjustment to the tooth, and asks you to close again. Then he smiles and says, "There. That should feel better." You get up, thank him, and leave. You feel a little tired, but calm and relaxed.

Index